BASIC TRAUMA LIFE SUPPORT FOR PARAMEDICS PROVIDER MANUAL
A COMPREHENSIVE GUIDE COVERING THE LATEST GUIDELINES

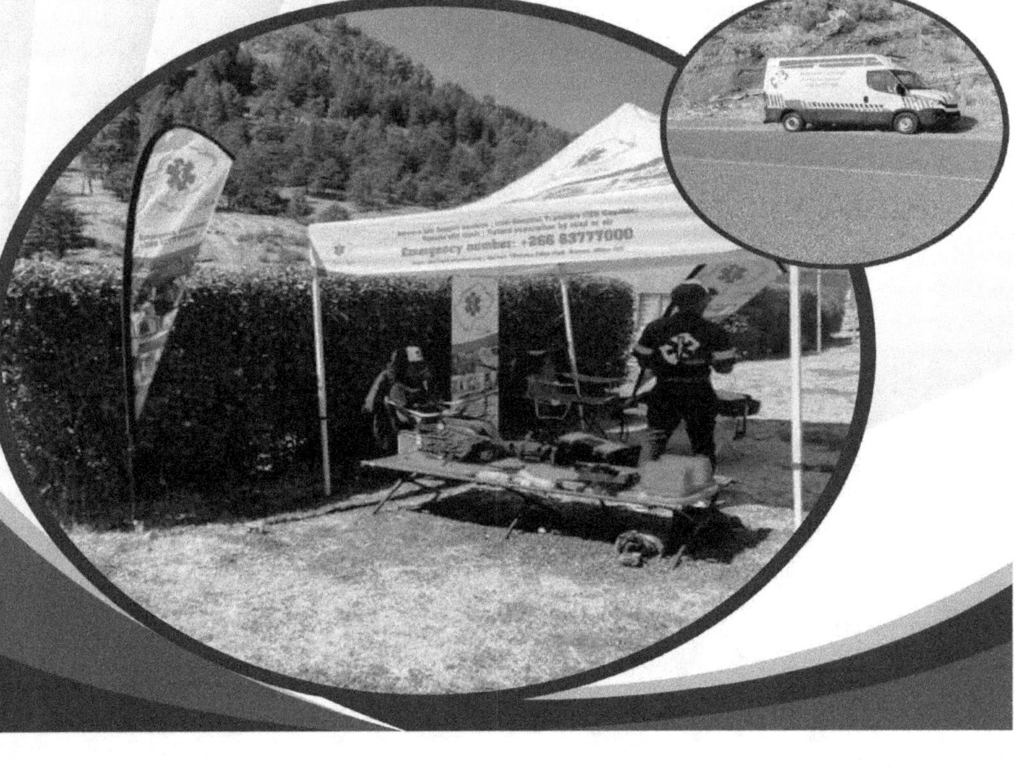

Author

Miss Evelin Limakatso Kholeli

Table of contents

1. Introduction to basic life support
2. Assessing the scene and patient
3. CPR for adults
4. CPR for children and infants
5. Using an automated external defibrillator
6. Special considerations
7. Legal and ethical considerations
8. Team-based BLS
9. Practical skills and scenarios
10. Post-resuscitation care

Introduction to Basic Life Support (BLS) Course

Welcome to the Basic Life Support (BLS) Course!

In emergency situations, timely and effective intervention can make the difference between life and death. The Basic Life Support (BLS) course is designed to equip individuals with essential skills and knowledge to manage critical emergencies until professional medical help arrives.

Purpose of the Course

The primary goal of this course is to provide you with the tools and confidence to perform life-saving techniques in various emergency scenarios. You will learn how to:

- **Assess** and prioritize patients' needs in life-threatening situations.
- **Perform Cardiopulmonary Resuscitation (CPR)** to help individuals who have stopped breathing or whose heart has stopped beating.
- **Use an Automated External Defibrillator (AED)** to deliver an electric shock to the heart in cases of cardiac arrest.
- **Manage Airway Obstruction** and ensure that the airway remains clear for effective breathing.
- **Provide Basic First Aid** to address common injuries and medical emergencies.

What You Will Learn

Throughout the course, you will gain hands-on experience and theoretical knowledge in:

- **Assessing the patient's condition**: Recognizing signs of respiratory and cardiac emergencies.
- **Performing effective CPR**: Understanding the correct compression and ventilation techniques for adults, children, and infants.
- **Using airway management tools**: Techniques for clearing and maintaining an open airway.
- **Operating an AED**: Steps for using an AED to assist in cardiac arrest situations.

- **Managing choking and other emergencies**: Strategies for handling airway obstructions and providing basic first aid.

Course Structure

The BLS course combines interactive lectures, practical demonstrations, and hands-on practice to ensure that you are well-prepared to respond in real-life situations. Certification is awarded upon successful completion, which not only validates your skills but also enhances your readiness to act in emergencies.

By the end of this course, you will be equipped with the confidence and competence to provide essential life support, potentially saving lives and making a significant impact in emergency situations.

We are excited to have you on this journey to becoming a skilled responder and making a difference when it matters most.

A Basic Life Support (BLS) course is designed for a wide range of individuals who may need to provide initial care in emergency situations. The course is suitable for:

1. Healthcare Professionals

- **Paramedics and EMTs**: Essential for those providing pre-hospital emergency care.
- **Nurses and Doctors**: Required for those working in various medical settings to manage emergencies effectively.
- **Hospital Staff**: Includes respiratory therapists, laboratory technicians, and other allied health professionals who may encounter emergency situations.

2. Public Safety and Emergency Responders

- **Firefighters**: Often required to have BLS training as part of their emergency response duties.
- **Police Officers**: Beneficial for handling medical emergencies while on duty.

3. Workplace Safety Personnel

- **First Responders**: Individuals trained to handle emergencies in various environments, such as factory or office safety officers.
- **Occupational Health and Safety Professionals**: Those responsible for ensuring safety protocols are in place and adhered to in the workplace.

4. Educational and Childcare Providers

- **Teachers and School Staff**: Important for those who may need to respond to medical emergencies involving students.
- **Childcare Workers**: Ensures readiness to handle emergencies involving children.

5. Community Members and General Public

- **Parents and Caregivers**: Helpful for those responsible for the well-being of children or elderly family members.
- **Anyone Interested in Lifesaving Skills**: Individuals who wish to be prepared to assist in emergencies, even if they are not in a healthcare or safety role.

6. Special Populations

- **Athletes and Coaches**: Those involved in sports and physical activities who may need to respond to injuries or medical emergencies.
- **Volunteers**: Individuals involved in community service or volunteer organizations that might encounter medical emergencies.

Training Requirements

- **No Prerequisites**: Generally, BLS courses do not require any prior medical training or certification.
- **Age and Health**: Most courses are open to adults of various ages and health conditions, though some courses may have age restrictions or health considerations for practical exercises.

Benefits of BLS Training

- **Life-Saving Skills**: Provides the knowledge and skills to perform CPR, use an AED, and manage choking and other emergencies effectively.
- **Confidence and Preparedness**: Enhances confidence in handling emergencies and contributes to overall safety in various environments.
- **Certification**: Many BLS courses offer certification upon successful completion, which can be a valuable credential for various roles and professions.

Basic Life Support (BLS) is a foundational level of medical care used to assist individuals experiencing life-threatening emergencies. It is typically performed until the patient can receive full medical care at a hospital. BLS includes various techniques that can be used to maintain an open airway, support breathing, and preserve circulation without the use of advanced equipment. Here is an introduction to the key components of Basic Life Support:

Key Components of Basic Life Support:

1. **Scene Safety and Assessment:**
   - Ensure the scene is safe for both the rescuer and the victim.
   - Quickly assess the situation to understand what happened and determine the need for BLS.
2. **Recognition of Cardiac Arrest:**
   - Check for responsiveness by gently shaking the person and shouting.
   - Look for normal breathing and check the pulse for no more than 10 seconds. Agonal gasps are not normal breathing.
3. **Activation of Emergency Response System:**
   - Call for help immediately if the person is unresponsive.
   - If alone, call emergency services and retrieve an Automated External Defibrillator (AED) if available.
4. **High-Quality Chest Compressions:**
   - Place the heel of one hand on the center of the chest, with the other hand on top.
   - Perform compressions at a depth of at least 2 inches (5 cm) for adults, allowing the chest to fully recoil between compressions.
   - Compress at a rate of 100-120 compressions per minute.
5. **Airway Management:**
   - Open the airway using the head-tilt-chin-lift maneuver if no spinal injury is suspected.
   - Use the jaw-thrust maneuver if a spinal injury is suspected.
6. **Rescue Breathing:**
   - Provide rescue breaths using a barrier device or mouth-to-mouth if no advanced airway is present.

- Give 2 breaths after every 30 compressions (for adults), ensuring each breath lasts about 1 second and makes the chest rise visibly.
7. **Use of Automated External Defibrillator (AED):**
    - Turn on the AED and follow the prompts.
    - Attach the AED pads to the victim's bare chest as indicated.
    - Stand clear while the AED analyzes the heart rhythm.
    - Deliver a shock if advised by the AED and immediately resume CPR starting with chest compressions.
8. **Continuing Care:**
    - Continue cycles of 30 compressions and 2 breaths until emergency medical services arrive or the person shows signs of life.
    - If the person starts breathing normally but remains unresponsive, place them in the recovery position and monitor their condition.

Training and Certification:

To perform BLS effectively, it is essential to receive proper training and certification from recognized organizations such as the American Heart Association (AHA) or the Red Cross. These organizations offer courses that cover all aspects of BLS and provide hands-on practice with manikins and AED trainers.

Importance of Basic Life Support:

BLS is critical because it can significantly improve the chances of survival and recovery for individuals experiencing cardiac arrest, choking, drowning, or other life-threatening emergencies. Timely and effective BLS can prevent brain damage and increase the likelihood of a positive outcome until advanced medical care can be provided.

Assessing the scene and patient is a crucial first step in Basic Life Support (BLS). This ensures the safety of both the rescuer and the patient, and allows the rescuer to quickly identify the patient's condition and the necessary steps to take. Here are the detailed steps:

Assessing the Scene:

1. Scene Safety:
    - **Ensure Personal Safety:** Before approaching the patient, make sure the scene is safe for you and bystanders. Look for potential hazards such as traffic, fire, electrical dangers, or violent situations.
    - **Environmental Awareness:** Be aware of your surroundings. Ensure you are not putting yourself in harm's way.
2. Initial Assessment:
    - **Quick Scan:** Perform a quick scan of the area to understand what might have happened. Look for clues that could explain the patient's condition (e.g., fallen ladder, spilled medication, etc.).
    - **Bystander Information:** If there are bystanders, ask them what happened. They might provide valuable information about the patient's condition and the events leading up to the emergency.

Assessing the Patient:

1. Check for Responsiveness:
    - **Approach the Patient:** Gently tap the patient's shoulder and shout to see if they respond.
    - **Shout for Help:** If the patient does not respond, shout for help to alert others that you need assistance.
2. Activate Emergency Response System:
    - **Call for Help:** If you are alone, call emergency services yourself and get an Automated External Defibrillator (AED) if available.
    - **Delegate Tasks:** If others are present, ask someone specific to call emergency services and another person to retrieve an AED.
3. Check Breathing and Pulse:
    - **Position the Patient:** Ensure the patient is lying flat on their back on a firm surface.
    - **Open the Airway:** Use the head-tilt-chin-lift maneuver to open the airway if no spinal injury is suspected.
    - **Look, Listen, and Feel for Breathing:** Place your ear close to the patient's mouth and nose, look at the chest for

movement, listen for breath sounds, and feel for breath on your cheek.
- **Check the Pulse:** Check for a carotid pulse by placing two fingers on the side of the neck, just below the jawbone. Check for no more than 10 seconds.
- **Agonal Gasps:** Be aware that occasional gasping breaths (agonal gasps) are not normal breathing and require immediate intervention.

4. **Determine Next Steps:**
   - **No Breathing and No Pulse:** If the patient is not breathing and has no pulse, begin high-quality chest compressions immediately.
   - **Breathing but Unresponsive:** If the patient is breathing but unresponsive, place them in the recovery position and continue to monitor their breathing and pulse until help arrives.
   - **Pulse but No Breathing:** If the patient has a pulse but is not breathing, begin rescue breathing (1 breath every 5-6 seconds for adults).

Importance of Effective Assessment:

- **Quick and Accurate:** The faster and more accurately you can assess the scene and the patient, the quicker you can initiate BLS, which is critical for the patient's survival.
- **Safety First:** Ensuring the scene is safe prevents additional injuries to the rescuer or bystanders.
- **Prioritization:** Proper assessment helps prioritize actions, such as calling for help, retrieving an AED, or starting chest compressions.

By following these steps, you can ensure that you are providing the best possible care in an emergency situation while maintaining safety for everyone involved.

Cardiopulmonary Resuscitation (CPR) is a critical component of Basic Life Support (BLS) for adults. It involves a combination of chest compressions and rescue breaths to maintain circulation and oxygenation in a person who has experienced cardiac arrest. Here are the detailed steps for performing CPR on adults:

Steps for Performing CPR on Adults:

1. **Check for Responsiveness and Breathing:**
   - **Tap and Shout:** Gently tap the person's shoulders and shout to see if they respond.
   - **Assess Breathing:** Look for normal breathing. Occasional gasps are not considered normal breathing.
   - **Call for Help:** If the person is unresponsive and not breathing normally, shout for help and activate the emergency response system. Send someone to call emergency services and get an Automated External Defibrillator (AED).
2. **Start Chest Compressions:**
   - **Positioning:** Place the person on their back on a firm, flat surface. Kneel beside them.
   - **Hand Placement:** Place the heel of one hand on the center of the chest (on the lower half of the sternum). Place your other hand on top of the first hand, interlocking your fingers.
   - **Compression Technique:** Use your body weight to push straight down, compressing the chest at least 2 inches (5 cm). Allow the chest to fully recoil between compressions.
   - **Compression Rate:** Perform compressions at a rate of 100-120 compressions per minute.
3. **Open the Airway:**
   - **Head-Tilt-Chin-Lift:** If no spinal injury is suspected, use the head-tilt-chin-lift maneuver to open the airway. Place one hand on the forehead and the other hand under the chin, then gently tilt the head back.
4. **Give Rescue Breaths:**
   - **Mouth-to-Mouth:** Pinch the nose shut and cover the person's mouth with yours, creating an airtight seal.
   - **Breath Delivery:** Give 2 breaths, each lasting about 1 second, watching for chest rise. If the chest does not rise, reposition the head and try again.

- **Breath to Compression Ratio:** Continue with cycles of 30 chest compressions followed by 2 rescue breaths.

5. **Use an AED (if available):**
   - **Turn on the AED:** As soon as the AED arrives, turn it on and follow the voice prompts.
   - **Attach AED Pads:** Expose the person's chest and attach the AED pads as shown on the diagrams on the pads.
   - **Analyze Rhythm:** Ensure no one is touching the person while the AED analyzes the heart rhythm.
   - **Deliver Shock:** If the AED advises a shock, ensure everyone is clear of the person and press the shock button.
   - **Resume CPR:** Immediately resume CPR starting with chest compressions after the shock is delivered or if no shock is advised.
6. **Continue CPR:**
   - **Cycle Continuation:** Continue performing cycles of 30 compressions and 2 breaths until emergency medical services (EMS) take over, the person shows signs of life (such as movement, breathing, or coughing), or you are too exhausted to continue.

Key Points to Remember:

- **Minimize Interruptions:** Minimize interruptions in chest compressions to increase the chances of a positive outcome.
- **Compression Depth and Rate:** Ensure compressions are at the correct depth (at least 2 inches) and rate (100-120 per minute).
- **Full Recoil:** Allow the chest to fully recoil between compressions to maximize blood flow.
- **Effective Breaths:** Ensure each breath makes the chest rise. If an advanced airway is in place, give 1 breath every 6 seconds without pausing compressions.
- **AED Use:** Use the AED as soon as it is available and follow its prompts precisely.

Performing CPR correctly can significantly increase the chances of survival and recovery for individuals experiencing cardiac arrest.

Proper training and regular practice are essential to maintain proficiency in these life-saving skills.

Performing CPR on children and infants involves similar principles as adult CPR but with some key differences due to their smaller size and different anatomical structures. Here's a detailed guide for CPR on children (1 year to puberty) and infants (under 1 year):

CPR for Children (1 year to puberty):

1. **Check for Responsiveness and Breathing:**
   - **Tap and Shout:** Tap the child's shoulder and shout to check for responsiveness.
   - **Assess Breathing:** Look for normal breathing. Occasional gasps are not considered normal breathing.
   - **Call for Help:** If the child is unresponsive and not breathing or only gasping, shout for help and activate the emergency response system. If you are alone, perform CPR for about 2 minutes before calling emergency services and retrieving an Automated External Defibrillator (AED).
2. **Start Chest Compressions:**
   - **Positioning:** Place the child on their back on a firm, flat surface. Kneel beside them.
   - **Hand Placement:** Use one or two hands (depending on the size of the child) placed on the lower half of the sternum.
   - **Compression Technique:** Compress the chest about 2 inches (5 cm). Allow the chest to fully recoil between compressions.
   - **Compression Rate:** Perform compressions at a rate of 100-120 compressions per minute.
3. **Open the Airway:**
   - **Head-Tilt-Chin-Lift:** If no spinal injury is suspected, use the head-tilt-chin-lift maneuver to open the airway.
4. **Give Rescue Breaths:**
   - **Mouth-to-Mouth or Mouth-to-Nose:** Pinch the nose shut and cover the child's mouth with yours, or cover both the nose and mouth if using the mouth-to-nose technique.

- **Breath Delivery:** Give 2 breaths, each lasting about 1 second, watching for chest rise. If the chest does not rise, reposition the head and try again.
- **Breath to Compression Ratio:** Continue with cycles of 30 chest compressions followed by 2 rescue breaths. If two rescuers are present, use a ratio of 15 compressions to 2 breaths.

5. **Use an AED (if available):**
   - **Turn on the AED:** As soon as the AED arrives, turn it on and follow the voice prompts.
   - **Attach AED Pads:** Use pediatric AED pads if available. If not, use adult pads, ensuring they do not touch each other.
   - **Analyze Rhythm:** Ensure no one is touching the child while the AED analyzes the heart rhythm.
   - **Deliver Shock:** If the AED advises a shock, ensure everyone is clear of the child and press the shock button.
   - **Resume CPR:** Immediately resume CPR starting with chest compressions after the shock is delivered or if no shock is advised.

6. **Continue CPR:**
   - **Cycle Continuation:** Continue performing cycles of 30 compressions and 2 breaths (or 15 compressions and 2 breaths if two rescuers are present) until EMS takes over, the child shows signs of life, or you are too exhausted to continue.

CPR for Infants (under 1 year):

1. **Check for Responsiveness and Breathing:**
   - **Tap and Shout:** Tap the infant's foot or gently tap their shoulder and shout to check for responsiveness.
   - **Assess Breathing:** Look for normal breathing. Occasional gasps are not considered normal breathing.
   - **Call for Help:** If the infant is unresponsive and not breathing or only gasping, shout for help and activate the emergency response system. If you are alone, perform CPR for about 2 minutes before calling emergency services and retrieving an AED.

2. **Start Chest Compressions:**
   - **Positioning:** Place the infant on their back on a firm, flat surface. Kneel or stand beside them.
   - **Hand Placement:** Use two fingers placed just below the nipple line on the breastbone.
   - **Compression Technique:** Compress the chest about 1.5 inches (4 cm). Allow the chest to fully recoil between compressions.
   - **Compression Rate:** Perform compressions at a rate of 100-120 compressions per minute.
3. **Open the Airway:**
   - **Head-Tilt-Chin-Lift:** Use a gentle head-tilt-chin-lift maneuver to open the airway, being careful not to tilt the head too far back.
4. **Give Rescue Breaths:**
   - **Mouth-to-Mouth and Nose:** Cover the infant's mouth and nose with your mouth, creating an airtight seal.
   - **Breath Delivery:** Give 2 gentle breaths, each lasting about 1 second, watching for chest rise. If the chest does not rise, reposition the head and try again.
   - **Breath to Compression Ratio:** Continue with cycles of 30 chest compressions followed by 2 rescue breaths. If two rescuers are present, use a ratio of 15 compressions to 2 breaths.
5. **Use an AED (if available):**
   - **Turn on the AED:** As soon as the AED arrives, turn it on and follow the voice prompts.
   - **Attach AED Pads:** Use pediatric AED pads if available. If not, use adult pads placed appropriately for the infant's size, ensuring they do not touch each other.
   - **Analyze Rhythm:** Ensure no one is touching the infant while the AED analyzes the heart rhythm.
   - **Deliver Shock:** If the AED advises a shock, ensure everyone is clear of the infant and press the shock button.
   - **Resume CPR:** Immediately resume CPR starting with chest compressions after the shock is delivered or if no shock is advised.
6. **Continue CPR:**

- **Cycle Continuation:** Continue performing cycles of 30 compressions and 2 breaths (or 15 compressions and 2 breaths if two rescuers are present) until EMS takes over, the infant shows signs of life, or you are too exhausted to continue.

Key Points to Remember:

- **Minimize Interruptions:** Minimize interruptions in chest compressions to increase the chances of a positive outcome.
- **Compression Depth and Rate:** Ensure compressions are at the correct depth and rate.
- **Full Recoil:** Allow the chest to fully recoil between compressions to maximize blood flow.
- **Effective Breaths:** Ensure each breath makes the chest rise. If an advanced airway is in place, give 1 breath every 6 seconds without pausing compressions.
- **AED Use:** Use the AED as soon as it is available and follow its prompts precisely.

Proper training and regular practice are essential to maintain proficiency in performing CPR on children and infants.

Using an Automated External Defibrillator (AED) is a critical component of Basic Life Support (BLS) and can significantly increase the chances of survival for someone experiencing sudden cardiac arrest. Here is a step-by-step guide on how to use an AED:

Steps for Using an AED:

1. **Ensure Scene Safety:**
   - Before using an AED, ensure the scene is safe for both the rescuer and the patient.
2. **Turn on the AED:**
   - Open the AED case and turn on the device. Many AEDs will turn on automatically when the case is opened.
3. **Follow AED Prompts:**
   - The AED will provide voice prompts and visual instructions. Follow these instructions carefully.

4. **Expose the Patient's Chest:**
    - Remove any clothing or objects (such as jewelry) that may interfere with AED pad placement.
    - If the chest is wet, quickly dry it. If the chest is excessively hairy, some AEDs come with a razor to quickly shave the area where the pads will be placed.
5. **Attach AED Pads:**
    - Peel the backing off the AED pads and place them on the patient's bare chest as shown in the diagrams on the pads.
    - **For Adults:** Place one pad on the upper right side of the chest (below the collarbone) and the other pad on the lower left side of the chest (a few inches below the armpit).
    - **For Children and Infants:** Use pediatric AED pads if available. If pediatric pads are not available, use adult pads, ensuring they do not touch each other. For smaller children and infants, place one pad on the center of the chest and the other pad on the back between the shoulder blades.
6. **Ensure No One Is Touching the Patient:**
    - Before the AED analyzes the heart rhythm, make sure no one is touching the patient. This ensures an accurate analysis.
7. **Allow the AED to Analyze:**
    - The AED will analyze the heart rhythm and determine if a shock is needed. Ensure everyone is clear of the patient during this time.
8. **Deliver the Shock:**
    - If the AED advises a shock, make sure no one is touching the patient and loudly announce "Clear!" before pressing the shock button.
    - Press the shock button to deliver the shock as instructed by the AED.
9. **Resume CPR:**
    - Immediately after delivering the shock, or if no shock is advised, resume CPR starting with chest compressions.
    - Continue CPR for about 2 minutes (or 5 cycles of 30 compressions and 2 breaths) before the AED reanalyzes the heart rhythm.
10. **Repeat as Necessary:**

- Continue to follow the AED prompts, delivering shocks if advised, and performing CPR until emergency medical services (EMS) arrive and take over, the patient shows signs of life (such as movement, breathing, or coughing), or you are too exhausted to continue.

Key Points to Remember:

- **Stay Calm:** Follow the AED prompts calmly and carefully.
- **Proper Pad Placement:** Ensure AED pads are placed correctly to maximize effectiveness.
- **Clear Communication:** Clearly announce "Clear!" before delivering a shock to ensure no one is in contact with the patient.
- **CPR Continuation:** Resume CPR immediately after shock delivery or if no shock is advised. High-quality chest compressions are essential.
- **AED Readiness:** Ensure the AED is always ready to use, with charged batteries and attached pads. Regularly check the AED as part of your emergency preparedness plan.

Using an AED effectively can save lives, but it's important to receive proper training and practice regularly to maintain proficiency in these life-saving skills.

In Basic Life Support (BLS), there are several special considerations to keep in mind to ensure that care is tailored to the specific needs and conditions of different patients and situations. These considerations can affect how you perform CPR, use an AED, and provide other critical interventions. Here are some of the key special considerations:

Special Considerations in BLS:

1. **Drowning Victims:**
    - **Initial Rescue Breaths:** For drowning victims, provide 2 initial rescue breaths before starting chest compressions. This helps deliver oxygen to the lungs which might be filled with water.

- **Focus on Effective Ventilation:** Ensure effective ventilations as hypoxia (lack of oxygen) is the primary concern in drowning.

2. **Trauma Victims:**
   - **Spinal Precautions:** If trauma is suspected, especially with potential spinal injuries, use the jaw-thrust maneuver to open the airway instead of the head-tilt-chin-lift maneuver.
   - **Bleeding Control:** Control any severe external bleeding with direct pressure or a tourniquet if necessary, in conjunction with CPR if needed.

3. **Pregnant Women:**
   - **Manual Uterine Displacement:** If the pregnant woman is in cardiac arrest, manually displace the uterus to the left to relieve pressure on the inferior vena cava, improving blood return to the heart.
   - **Positioning:** Perform CPR with the patient slightly tilted to the left side if possible to avoid compressing the large blood vessels by the uterus.

4. **Hypothermia:**
   - **Gentle Handling:** Handle hypothermic patients gently to avoid triggering cardiac arrhythmias.
   - **Extended Resuscitation Efforts:** Resuscitation efforts may be prolonged because hypothermic patients can have a better chance of recovery with extended CPR and rewarming.

5. **Pacemakers and Implanted Defibrillators:**
   - **Pad Placement:** When using an AED, avoid placing pads directly over an implanted device. Place the pads at least an inch away from the device to ensure effective shock delivery.

6. **Children and Infants:**
   - **Different Techniques:** Use different techniques and equipment sizes (e.g., pediatric AED pads) suitable for children and infants.
   - **Compression Depth:** Ensure appropriate compression depth (about 2 inches for children, about 1.5 inches for infants) and compression-to-breath ratios (30:2 for single rescuer, 15:2 for two rescuers).

7. **Obstructed Airway:**

- **Conscious Patients:** For conscious patients with an obstructed airway, use abdominal thrusts (Heimlich maneuver) in adults and children, and back slaps and chest thrusts in infants.
- **Unconscious Patients:** For unconscious patients, start CPR. Each time you open the airway to give breaths, look for the obstructing object and remove it if visible.

8. **Opioid Overdose:**
   - **Naloxone Administration:** If opioid overdose is suspected, administer naloxone if available, in addition to standard BLS measures.
   - **Breathing Support:** Ensure effective ventilation, as respiratory arrest is common in opioid overdoses.

9. **Chest Trauma:**
   - **Avoid Excessive Ventilation Pressure:** Be cautious with ventilation to avoid exacerbating injuries such as pneumothorax (collapsed lung).
   - **Assessment and Treatment:** Look for signs of chest trauma, such as flail chest, and manage accordingly while continuing CPR if needed.

10. **Foreign Body Airway Obstruction:**
    - **Adult and Child:** For a conscious adult or child, use abdominal thrusts (Heimlich maneuver). If the person becomes unconscious, begin CPR and check the mouth for the obstructing object before giving breaths.
    - **Infant:** For a conscious infant, use a combination of 5 back blows followed by 5 chest thrusts. If the infant becomes unconscious, start CPR and look for the object each time you open the airway to give breaths.

General Principles:

- **Safety First:** Always ensure the scene is safe before approaching the patient.
- **Early Activation of Emergency Services:** Activate the emergency response system as soon as possible.
- **Minimize Interruptions:** Minimize interruptions in chest compressions to maintain blood flow.

- **Teamwork:** Coordinate with other rescuers effectively, especially when dealing with special considerations, to provide optimal care.

Being aware of these special considerations and adapting your BLS approach accordingly can improve patient outcomes in diverse emergency situations. Proper training and regular practice are essential to effectively incorporate these considerations into your BLS skills.

Legal and ethical considerations in Basic Life Support (BLS) are crucial for ensuring that care is provided in a manner that respects the rights and safety of both the patient and the rescuer. Here are some key points to keep in mind:

Legal Considerations:

1. **Good Samaritan Laws:**
   - **Protection for Rescuers:** Good Samaritan laws protect individuals who provide reasonable assistance to those who are injured, ill, in peril, or otherwise incapacitated. These laws vary by jurisdiction but generally offer legal protection from liability as long as the rescuer acts in good faith and within their level of training.
   - **Limitations:** The protection does not cover gross negligence or willful misconduct.
2. **Duty to Act:**
   - **Professional Rescuers:** Certain professionals, such as paramedics, nurses, and doctors, have a duty to act when they are on duty. This duty requires them to provide care according to their training and scope of practice.
   - **Lay Rescuers:** Laypersons typically do not have a legal duty to provide aid unless a pre-existing duty exists, such as a parent-child relationship or in some employment situations.
3. **Consent:**
   - **Implied Consent:** In emergencies where the patient is unconscious, unresponsive, or unable to give consent, it is generally assumed that the patient would consent to life-saving interventions.

- **Informed Consent:** When the patient is conscious and capable of making decisions, obtaining informed consent before providing care is necessary. Explain what you intend to do and seek their agreement.

4. **Refusal of Care:**
    - **Respecting Wishes:** If a competent adult refuses care, you must respect their wishes, even if you disagree with their decision. Ensure that the refusal is documented and, if possible, witnessed.
    - **Documentation:** Document the patient's refusal of care, including their reasons and any discussions that took place.

5. **Confidentiality:**
    - **Patient Privacy:** Protect the patient's privacy by only sharing information with those directly involved in their care. This includes medical personnel and, when necessary, emergency contacts.
    - **HIPAA Compliance:** Follow regulations such as the Health Insurance Portability and Accountability Act (HIPAA) in the United States to safeguard patient information.

Ethical Considerations:

1. **Beneficence:**
    - **Acting in the Patient's Best Interest:** Always aim to do good and act in the best interest of the patient. Provide care that is intended to benefit the patient and improve their condition.

2. **Non-Maleficence:**
    - **Avoiding Harm:** Do no harm. Ensure that the care you provide does not harm the patient. This includes performing procedures correctly and within your level of training.

3. **Autonomy:**
    - **Respecting Patient Autonomy:** Respect the patient's right to make decisions about their own care. This includes honoring their wishes and advance directives, such as Do Not Resuscitate (DNR) orders.
    - **Informed Decision-Making:** Ensure that patients are fully informed about their condition and the proposed interventions so they can make autonomous decisions.

4. **Justice:**
    - **Fair and Equitable Care:** Provide care fairly and without discrimination. Treat all patients with respect and dignity, regardless of their background, status, or personal characteristics.
5. **Fidelity:**
    - **Honesty and Integrity:** Be honest with patients and their families. Maintain integrity in your actions and communications. Keep promises and commitments made to patients and colleagues.
6. **Cultural Sensitivity:**
    - **Respecting Cultural Differences:** Be aware of and respect cultural differences that may affect a patient's preferences and decisions regarding their care.

Practical Application:

1. **Training and Competence:**
    - **Stay Current:** Ensure that your training is up-to-date and that you are competent in the skills you may need to use in an emergency.
    - **Know Your Limits:** Act within the scope of your training and knowledge. Do not perform procedures you are not trained to do.
2. **Communication:**
    - **Clear and Compassionate:** Communicate clearly, compassionately, and respectfully with patients and their families.
    - **Documentation:** Accurately document all care provided, including the patient's condition, interventions performed, and the patient's response.
3. **Ethical Dilemmas:**
    - **Seek Guidance:** In situations where ethical dilemmas arise, seek guidance from colleagues, supervisors, or ethical committees if available.
    - **Reflect on Decisions:** Reflect on your decisions and actions to continuously improve your ethical practice.

Understanding and adhering to these legal and ethical principles ensures that BLS providers deliver care responsibly, respecting both the law and the dignity of the patients they serve.

Team-based Basic Life Support (BLS) is a collaborative approach to emergency care where multiple rescuers work together to provide effective and efficient care. Effective teamwork can improve patient outcomes by ensuring that each team member performs their role optimally. Here are some key aspects of team-based BLS:

Roles and Responsibilities:

1. **Team Leader:**
   - **Coordination:** The team leader coordinates all activities, making critical decisions and ensuring that all team members are aware of their roles and tasks.
   - **Communication:** The team leader communicates clearly and directs the team, giving specific instructions and providing feedback.
2. **Compressor:**
   - **Chest Compressions:** The primary role of the compressor is to perform high-quality chest compressions, maintaining a rate of 100-120 compressions per minute and a depth of at least 2 inches (5 cm) for adults, about 2 inches for children, and about 1.5 inches (4 cm) for infants.
   - **Rotation:** Compressors should rotate every 2 minutes (or sooner if fatigued) to maintain the quality of compressions. The team leader ensures smooth transitions.
3. **Airway Manager:**
   - **Airway Maintenance:** The airway manager is responsible for maintaining a patent airway, using techniques such as the head-tilt-chin-lift or jaw-thrust maneuver.
   - **Ventilations:** Provide rescue breaths using a bag-valve-mask (BVM) device, ensuring each breath lasts about 1 second and makes the chest rise. For infants and small children, provide breaths using the appropriate size mask.
   - **Advanced Airway:** If an advanced airway device (e.g., endotracheal tube) is available and within the scope of

practice, the airway manager may assist in its placement and secure it.
4. **AED/Monitor/Defibrillator Operator:**
   - **AED Operation:** The AED operator is responsible for applying the AED pads, turning on the device, and following the prompts.
   - **Shock Delivery:** Ensure that no one is touching the patient before delivering a shock. The operator also announces "Clear!" to ensure safety.
   - **Rhythm Analysis:** Regularly analyze the heart rhythm as directed by the AED or monitor.
5. **IV/IO Medication Administrator:**
   - **Medication Administration:** If within the scope of practice, this team member establishes IV or IO access and administers medications as directed by protocols or the team leader.
   - **Documentation:** Document all medications administered, including time, dosage, and patient response.
6. **Recorder:**
   - **Documentation:** The recorder keeps a detailed log of events, including the time of interventions, medications given, and patient responses.
   - **Support:** Provides additional support as needed, such as preparing equipment or assisting other team members.

Key Elements of Effective Team-Based BLS:

1. **Clear Communication:**
   - **Closed-Loop Communication:** Use closed-loop communication to ensure messages are heard and understood. The sender gives instructions, the receiver repeats them back, and the sender confirms.
   - **Concise Commands:** The team leader gives clear, concise commands to avoid confusion.
2. **Role Clarity:**
   - **Defined Roles:** Each team member should know their specific role and responsibilities. This clarity helps in efficient task execution and reduces overlap.

- **Role Assignment:** The team leader assigns roles based on the team members' skills and training.
3. **Effective Coordination:**
    - **Task Delegation:** The team leader delegates tasks effectively, ensuring that all aspects of care are covered.
    - **Smooth Transitions:** Ensure smooth transitions between tasks, such as switching compressors every 2 minutes.
4. **Situational Awareness:**
    - **Monitor the Patient:** Continuously monitor the patient's condition and be prepared to adjust interventions as needed.
    - **Environmental Awareness:** Be aware of the environment to ensure safety and efficiency. This includes ensuring a clear space for CPR and AED use.
5. **Mutual Support:**
    - **Assistance:** Team members should assist each other as needed, recognizing signs of fatigue or difficulty.
    - **Backup:** Provide backup and support to ensure continuous high-quality care.
6. **Debriefing:**
    - **Post-Event Debrief:** After the event, conduct a debriefing session to review performance, identify areas for improvement, and provide feedback.
    - **Continuous Improvement:** Use debriefing to continuously improve team performance and patient outcomes.

Practical Steps for Implementing Team-Based BLS:

1. **Training and Practice:**
    - **Regular Drills:** Conduct regular team-based BLS drills to practice roles and improve coordination.
    - **Scenario-Based Training:** Use scenario-based training to simulate real-life emergencies and practice team dynamics.
2. **Equipment Familiarity:**
    - **Know Your Tools:** Ensure all team members are familiar with the equipment, such as AEDs, BVMs, and advanced airway devices.
    - **Quick Access:** Ensure all equipment is easily accessible and ready for use.

3. **Standard Operating Procedures:**
    - **Protocols:** Develop and follow standard operating procedures for team-based BLS to ensure consistency and high-quality care.
    - **Guidelines:** Follow established guidelines and protocols, such as those from the American Heart Association (AHA) or equivalent organizations.

Effective team-based BLS relies on clear communication, defined roles, coordinated actions, and continuous practice. By working together efficiently, a BLS team can significantly improve the chances of survival and positive outcomes for patients experiencing cardiac arrest or other life-threatening emergencies.

Practical skills and scenario-based training are crucial components of Basic Life Support (BLS) education. These skills help ensure that rescuers are prepared to respond effectively in real-life emergencies. Below are some essential BLS skills and scenarios that can be practiced to enhance proficiency and readiness.

Essential BLS Skills

1. **High-Quality CPR:**
    - **Chest Compressions:**
        - **Adults:** Compress the chest at least 2 inches (5 cm) deep at a rate of 100-120 compressions per minute.
        - **Children:** Compress the chest about 2 inches (5 cm) deep.
        - **Infants:** Compress the chest about 1.5 inches (4 cm) deep.
        - **Recoil:** Allow the chest to fully recoil between compressions.
    - **Ventilations:**
        - Give 2 rescue breaths after every 30 compressions (or after every 15 compressions if two rescuers are present for a child or infant).
        - Each breath should last about 1 second and cause visible chest rise.
2. **Using an AED:**

- Pad Placement:
  - **Adults:** Place one pad on the upper right side of the chest and the other on the lower left side.
  - **Children/Infants:** Use pediatric pads if available; if not, place adult pads ensuring they do not touch.
- Operation:
  - Turn on the AED and follow the prompts.
  - Ensure no one is touching the patient during rhythm analysis and shock delivery.

3. Airway Management:
   - **Head-Tilt-Chin-Lift:** Use this technique to open the airway in patients without suspected spinal injury.
   - **Jaw-Thrust:** Use this technique to open the airway in patients with suspected spinal injury.
   - **Bag-Valve-Mask (BVM):** Properly use a BVM to deliver effective breaths.

4. Foreign Body Airway Obstruction:
   - **Conscious Adult/Child:** Perform abdominal thrusts (Heimlich maneuver).
   - **Conscious Infant:** Perform a combination of 5 back blows and 5 chest thrusts.
   - **Unconscious Patient:** Begin CPR and look for the object each time you open the airway to give breaths.

Scenario-Based Training

1. **Cardiac Arrest in an Adult:**
   - **Scenario:** An adult collapses and is unresponsive.
   - **Actions:**
     - Ensure scene safety.
     - Check for responsiveness and breathing.
     - Call for help and activate the emergency response system.
     - Start CPR and use an AED as soon as it arrives.
2. **Cardiac Arrest in a Child:**
   - **Scenario:** A child is found unresponsive in a park.
   - **Actions:**
     - Ensure scene safety.

- Check for responsiveness and breathing.
- Shout for help and send someone to call emergency services.
- Start CPR with a 30:2 compression-to-breath ratio (or 15:2 if two rescuers are present).
- Use an AED as soon as it arrives.

3. **Cardiac Arrest in an Infant:**
    - **Scenario:** An infant is found unresponsive in a crib.
    - **Actions:**
        - Ensure scene safety.
        - Check for responsiveness and breathing.
        - Shout for help and call emergency services.
        - Start CPR with a 30:2 compression-to-breath ratio (or 15:2 if two rescuers are present).
        - Use an AED with pediatric pads if available.

4. **Drowning Victim:**
    - **Scenario:** A person is pulled from a swimming pool, unresponsive and not breathing.
    - **Actions:**
        - Ensure scene safety.
        - Provide 2 initial rescue breaths before starting chest compressions.
        - Call for help and activate the emergency response system.
        - Continue CPR and use an AED as soon as it arrives.

5. **Trauma Victim with Suspected Spinal Injury:**
    - **Scenario:** A person falls from a height and is unresponsive with suspected spinal injury.
    - **Actions:**
        - Ensure scene safety.
        - Use the jaw-thrust maneuver to open the airway.
        - Call for help and activate the emergency response system.
        - Start CPR if there are no signs of life and use an AED as soon as it arrives.

6. **Choking Adult:**
    - **Scenario:** An adult is choking and cannot speak or breathe.
    - **Actions:**

- Ask if they are choking and need help.
- Perform abdominal thrusts until the object is expelled or the person becomes unresponsive.
- If unresponsive, start CPR and look for the object each time you open the airway to give breaths.

7. **Choking Infant:**
   - **Scenario:** An infant is choking and cannot cry or breathe.
   - **Actions:**
     - Perform 5 back blows followed by 5 chest thrusts.
     - If the infant becomes unresponsive, start CPR and look for the object each time you open the airway to give breaths.

Implementing Practical Skills and Scenarios

1. **Regular Practice:**
   - Schedule regular practice sessions to keep skills sharp.
   - Use mannequins and simulation tools to create realistic scenarios.
2. **Team Drills:**
   - Practice team-based BLS scenarios to improve coordination and communication.
   - Rotate roles to ensure all team members are proficient in each task.
3. **Feedback and Debriefing:**
   - Conduct debriefing sessions after each practice scenario to discuss what went well and areas for improvement.
   - Provide constructive feedback to all participants.
4. **Continuous Education:**
   - Stay updated with the latest guidelines and protocols from organizations like the American Heart Association (AHA).
   - Attend refresher courses and advanced training sessions as needed.

By regularly practicing these skills and scenarios, BLS providers can ensure they are well-prepared to respond effectively in real-life emergencies, ultimately improving patient outcomes.

Post-resuscitation care is a critical phase that follows successful return of spontaneous circulation (ROSC) after cardiac arrest. The goal of post-resuscitation care is to stabilize the patient, optimize organ function, and prevent further complications. Here are the key components of post-resuscitation care in BLS:

Key Components of Post-Resuscitation Care:

1. **Airway and Breathing Management:**
    - **Maintain Airway Patency:** Ensure the airway remains open. Use airway adjuncts if necessary, such as oropharyngeal or nasopharyngeal airways.
    - **Adequate Ventilation and Oxygenation:** Provide oxygen to maintain an oxygen saturation (SpO2) of 94-99%. Use bag-valve-mask (BVM) ventilation if needed.
    - **Monitor Respiratory Effort:** Watch for signs of respiratory distress and provide support as needed. Be prepared to assist with advanced airway management if within your scope of practice.
2. **Circulation and Hemodynamic Stabilization:**
    - **Monitor Vital Signs:** Continuously monitor heart rate, blood pressure, and oxygen saturation.
    - **IV/IO Access:** Ensure intravenous (IV) or intraosseous (IO) access is established for fluid administration and medications.
    - **Fluid Resuscitation:** Administer fluids as needed to maintain adequate blood pressure and perfusion.
    - **Medications:** Administer medications as directed by advanced life support protocols or a medical provider.
3. **Neurological Support:**
    - **Assess Level of Consciousness:** Regularly assess the patient's level of consciousness using tools like the Glasgow Coma Scale (GCS).
    - **Temperature Management:** Prevent hyperthermia by ensuring the patient does not become overheated. If indicated, initiate targeted temperature management (therapeutic hypothermia) to improve neurological

outcomes. This is typically initiated by advanced life support providers.
4. **Transport and Handoff:**
    - **Prepare for Transport:** Ensure the patient is stable for transport to a higher level of care, such as a hospital with advanced cardiac care capabilities.
    - **Communicate with Receiving Facility:** Provide a detailed report to the receiving medical facility, including the patient's history, the events leading to the cardiac arrest, the interventions performed, and the patient's response to those interventions.
5. **Continuous Monitoring:**
    - **ECG Monitoring:** Continuously monitor the patient's cardiac rhythm to detect any arrhythmias or recurrence of cardiac arrest.
    - **Frequent Reassessment:** Regularly reassess the patient's condition, including vital signs, neurological status, and overall stability.
6. **Documentation:**
    - **Detailed Record-Keeping:** Document all care provided, including the times of interventions, medications administered, and the patient's response. Accurate documentation is crucial for ongoing care and legal purposes.

Practical Steps for Post-Resuscitation Care:

1. **Initial Stabilization:**
    - **Ensure ROSC:** Confirm that the patient has achieved return of spontaneous circulation (ROSC).
    - **Secure Airway:** Ensure the patient's airway is secure and they are receiving adequate oxygenation and ventilation.
2. **Monitoring and Support:**
    - **Vital Signs Monitoring:** Continuously monitor vital signs, including heart rate, blood pressure, and oxygen saturation.
    - **Fluid and Medication Administration:** Administer fluids and medications as needed to stabilize the patient's hemodynamic status.

3. **Prepare for Transport:**
    - **Stable for Transport:** Ensure the patient is stable for transport to a hospital or advanced care facility.
    - **Communication:** Provide a thorough handoff to the receiving medical team, including all relevant patient information and the interventions performed.
4. **Collaborate with Advanced Life Support Providers:**
    - **ALS Support:** Work closely with advanced life support (ALS) providers, who can provide advanced airway management, more complex medications, and further diagnostic and therapeutic interventions.
5. **Reassessment and Adjustment:**
    - **Continuous Reassessment:** Regularly reassess the patient's condition and adjust care as needed based on their response.
    - **Adapt to Changes:** Be prepared to adapt to changes in the patient's condition, including potential re-arrest or deterioration.

Scenario Example: Post-Resuscitation Care in Practice

Scenario:

You and your team successfully resuscitate a 60-year-old male who collapsed and was found unresponsive with no pulse. After several minutes of high-quality CPR and one shock from the AED, ROSC is achieved.

Actions:

1. **Airway and Breathing:**
    - Ensure the patient's airway is open and clear.
    - Administer high-flow oxygen via a non-rebreather mask or BVM.
    - Monitor respiratory rate and effort, providing ventilatory support if needed.
2. **Circulation:**
    - Establish IV access and begin fluid resuscitation as needed.
    - Continuously monitor heart rate and blood pressure.

- Administer medications as directed by advanced protocols or a medical provider.

3. **Neurological:**
    - Assess the patient's level of consciousness using the GCS.
    - Implement measures to prevent hyperthermia and consider initiating targeted temperature management if indicated.
4. **Transport Preparation:**
    - Prepare the patient for transport to the nearest hospital with advanced cardiac care capabilities.
    - Communicate with the receiving facility, providing a detailed report of the patient's status and interventions performed.
5. **Documentation:**
    - Document all actions taken, including the time of ROSC, medications administered, and the patient's response.
6. **Handoff:**
    - Provide a comprehensive handoff to the receiving medical team, ensuring they have all the necessary information to continue care.

By following these steps, you can ensure that the patient receives high-quality post-resuscitation care, improving their chances of survival and recovery. Regular training and scenario-based practice can help you and your team stay prepared for these critical situations.

Checking scene safety and performing a thorough assessment are crucial first steps in Basic Life Support (BLS) to ensure that both the rescuer and the patient are protected and to provide effective care. Here's a step-by-step guide to checking scene safety and performing an initial assessment:

Steps to Check Scene Safety and Assessment in BLS

1. Check Scene Safety

1. **Assess the Environment:**
    - **Look for Hazards:** Quickly scan the scene for any immediate dangers such as traffic, fire, electrical hazards, hazardous materials, or unstable structures.

- **Evaluate the Area:** Ensure that the area is safe for you and the patient. If there are dangers, take steps to mitigate them if possible or move to a safer location if it's safe to do so.
2. **Protect Yourself:**
    - **Use Personal Protective Equipment (PPE):** If available, use gloves, masks, and other PPE to protect yourself from potential exposure to bodily fluids or infections.
    - **Ensure Safety of Others:** If there are bystanders, ensure they are kept away from the danger zone to prevent additional casualties.
3. **Identify the Cause of the Incident:**
    - **Assess Mechanism of Injury:** If applicable, determine how the patient was injured (e.g., car accident, fall) to understand potential injuries and take appropriate precautions.

2. Initial Assessment of the Patient

1. **Determine Responsiveness:**
    - **Tap and Shout:** Gently tap the patient and shout, "Are you okay?" or "Can you hear me?" to check if they are responsive.
    - **Look for Movement:** Observe if the patient moves, opens their eyes, or makes any sounds in response to your stimuli.
2. **Call for Help:**
    - **Activate Emergency Services:** If the patient is unresponsive or in need of assistance, immediately call for emergency medical services (EMS). If you are alone, activate the emergency response system by calling 911 (or the local emergency number) and provide details about the location and nature of the emergency.
3. **Assess Breathing:**
    - **Look, Listen, and Feel:** Check for breathing by looking for chest rise and fall, listening for breath sounds, and feeling for breath on your cheek.
    - **Check for Normal Breathing:** Assess for normal breathing for no more than 10 seconds. If the patient is not breathing

or has abnormal breathing (e.g., gasping), proceed to the next steps.
4. **Check Pulse (if trained):**
    - **Locate Pulse Points:** For adults, check the carotid pulse on the side of the neck. For infants, check the brachial pulse on the inside of the upper arm.
    - **Assess Pulse:** Check for the presence of a pulse for no more than 10 seconds. If you cannot feel a pulse, or if it is very weak or irregular, initiate CPR.
5. **Assess for Severe Bleeding:**
    - **Look for Visible Blood Loss:** Check the patient's body for signs of severe external bleeding.
    - **Apply Pressure:** If there is severe bleeding, apply direct pressure to the wound to control it.
6. **Position the Patient:**
    - **If Breathing and Responsive:** If the patient is breathing and responsive, place them in the recovery position (on their side) to maintain an open airway and prevent choking.
    - **If Unresponsive and Not Breathing:** If the patient is unresponsive and not breathing, start CPR immediately.
7. **Perform CPR if Necessary:**
    - **Start CPR:** Begin chest compressions and rescue breaths according to the BLS guidelines if the patient is unresponsive and not breathing normally.
8. **Use an AED if Available:**
    - **Apply AED Pads:** Follow the AED's prompts if an automated external defibrillator (AED) is available. Ensure that no one is touching the patient when the AED is analyzing or delivering a shock.

Summary of Key Points:

- **Ensure Scene Safety:** Quickly evaluate and secure the scene to ensure it is safe for you and the patient.
- **Check Responsiveness:** Determine if the patient is responsive by using verbal and physical stimuli.
- **Activate EMS:** Call for emergency medical assistance if needed.

- **Assess Breathing and Pulse:** Check for breathing and pulse to determine if CPR is required.
- **Control Bleeding:** Look for and control severe bleeding if present.
- **Position and Care:** Place the patient in the recovery position if responsive and breathing; initiate CPR if unresponsive and not breathing.

These initial steps are critical in the BLS process to ensure that you provide appropriate and effective care while maintaining your own safety and the safety of others. Regular practice and training help to ensure that these steps are performed quickly and efficiently in real-life emergencies.

Recognizing cardiac arrest is crucial for initiating appropriate Basic Life Support (BLS) interventions. Cardiac arrest occurs when the heart suddenly stops beating effectively, leading to a lack of blood flow to vital organs. Here's how to recognize cardiac arrest:

Key Indicators of Cardiac Arrest

1. **Unresponsiveness:**
   - **Check Responsiveness:** Gently tap the patient and shout, "Are you okay?" or "Can you hear me?" If the patient does not respond to verbal or physical stimuli, they are likely unresponsive.
   - **Lack of Movement:** An unresponsive patient will not make purposeful movements or react to stimuli.
2. **Absence of Normal Breathing:**
   - **Look, Listen, and Feel:** Assess the patient's breathing by looking for chest rise, listening for breath sounds, and feeling for breath on your cheek.
   - **Check for Abnormal Breathing:** If the patient is not breathing or is only gasping (agonal breathing), this is a sign of cardiac arrest or a life-threatening emergency.
   - **Normal Breathing:** Normal breathing includes regular, effortless breaths. If breathing is absent or abnormal, proceed with further steps.
3. **Absence of a Pulse (if trained):**

- **Check Pulse:** For adults, check the carotid pulse on the side of the neck. For infants, check the brachial pulse on the inside of the upper arm.
- **Assess for Pulse:** Use your fingers to feel for the pulse. You should check for no more than 10 seconds. If no pulse is detected or if it is very weak, initiate CPR.

Steps to Recognize Cardiac Arrest

1. **Assess the Scene:**
   - Ensure the scene is safe before approaching the patient.
2. **Check Responsiveness:**
   - Tap and shout to check if the patient is responsive.
3. **Check for Breathing:**
   - Look for chest rise and fall.
   - Listen for breath sounds.
   - Feel for breath on your cheek.
4. **Check for Pulse:**
   - For adults, check the carotid pulse.
   - For infants, check the brachial pulse.
   - Do this for no more than 10 seconds.
5. **Determine Cardiac Arrest:**
   - If the patient is unresponsive, not breathing normally, and has no detectable pulse, this indicates cardiac arrest.

Immediate Actions After Recognition

1. **Call for Help:**
   - Activate the emergency response system by calling 911 (or the local emergency number) and provide details about the situation.
2. **Start CPR:**
   - **Chest Compressions:** Begin chest compressions at a rate of 100-120 compressions per minute and a depth of at least 2 inches (5 cm) for adults. For children and infants, adjust the depth accordingly.
   - **Rescue Breaths:** Provide 2 rescue breaths after every 30 compressions (or 15 compressions if two rescuers are present for a child or infant).

3. **Use an AED (if available):**
   - **Apply AED Pads:** Follow the AED's prompts to analyze the heart rhythm and deliver a shock if advised.
   - **Follow Prompts:** Ensure no one is touching the patient during analysis or shock delivery.
4. **Continue Care:**
   - **Ongoing CPR:** Continue CPR until emergency medical services arrive, the patient shows signs of life, or you are too exhausted to continue.

By quickly recognizing the signs of cardiac arrest and initiating BLS, you can improve the chances of survival for the patient. Regular training and practice help to ensure that these steps are performed effectively in real emergencies.

Activating the emergency response system is a crucial step in Basic Life Support (BLS) that ensures professional medical help is on the way. Here's how to activate the emergency response system effectively:

Steps to Activate the Emergency Response System

1. Assess the Situation

- **Determine the Need:** Confirm that emergency medical assistance is needed by checking the patient's responsiveness, breathing, and pulse. If the patient is unresponsive and not breathing normally (or has no pulse), or if there is a life-threatening condition, you need to activate the emergency response system.

2. Call for Help

- **Determine the Communication Method:**
   - **Direct Communication:** If you are in a location with a landline or mobile phone, use it to call emergency services directly.
   - **Send a Bystander:** If you are alone with the patient, you can call emergency services yourself if you have a mobile phone. If there are other people around, send someone else to make the call while you provide care.

- Dial the Emergency Number:
    - **In the United States:** Dial 911.
    - **In other countries:** Use the local emergency number (e.g., 112 in many European countries, 000 in Australia).

3. Provide Essential Information

- **Identify Yourself:**
    - State your name and location clearly so the dispatcher knows where to send help.
- **Explain the Situation:**
    - Describe the emergency situation concisely, including what happened and the condition of the patient.
- **Provide Specific Details:**
    - **Location:** Give the exact address or location of the incident.
    - **Number of Patients:** Indicate how many people are affected.
    - **Condition of the Patient:** Mention if the patient is unresponsive, not breathing, or has no pulse.
    - **Any Hazards:** Inform the dispatcher of any potential hazards or dangers at the scene (e.g., fire, traffic, chemicals).
- **Follow Instructions:**
    - Listen to the dispatcher's instructions and follow them carefully. They may provide guidance on immediate actions to take until help arrives.

4. Continue Providing Care

- **Resume Care:** While waiting for emergency services, continue to provide BLS care, such as CPR and using an AED, if indicated.
- **Stay on the Line:** If you're on the phone with emergency services, stay on the line until instructed to hang up. Provide any additional information requested by the dispatcher.

5. Prepare for Arrival of EMS

- **Clear the Area:** Make sure the area around the patient is clear and accessible for emergency responders.

- **Meet the Responders:** If possible, go to the entrance of the location or send someone to guide the emergency medical team to the patient.

Tips for Effective Communication

- **Stay Calm:** Keep a clear and calm demeanor to ensure effective communication with the dispatcher.
- **Be Concise:** Provide information in a clear and concise manner to avoid confusion.
- **Verify Details:** If you are unsure about any details, it's better to verify them with the dispatcher than to provide incorrect information.

By following these steps, you can effectively activate the emergency response system, ensuring that professional medical help arrives as quickly as possible.

High-quality chest compressions are a critical component of effective CPR (cardiopulmonary resuscitation) and significantly increase the chances of survival in cardiac arrest cases. Here's a guide to performing high-quality chest compressions according to BLS (Basic Life Support) guidelines:

Key Components of High-Quality Chest Compressions

1. **Depth of Compressions:**
   - **Adults:** Compress the chest at least 2 inches (5 cm) deep.
   - **Children:** Compress the chest about 2 inches (5 cm) deep.
   - **Infants:** Compress the chest about 1.5 inches (4 cm) deep.
2. **Rate of Compressions:**
   - Perform chest compressions at a rate of 100-120 compressions per minute.
3. **Allow Complete Chest Recoil:**
   - Ensure that the chest fully recoils between compressions. This allows the heart to refill with blood, improving the effectiveness of each compression.
4. **Minimize Interruptions:**

- Avoid interruptions in chest compressions as much as possible. Continuous compressions are crucial for maintaining blood flow to vital organs.

5. **Proper Hand Placement:**
    - **Adults:** Place the heel of one hand on the center of the chest, on the lower half of the sternum. Place the other hand on top and interlock the fingers.
    - **Children:** Use one or two hands (depending on the size of the child) to perform compressions, placing them on the center of the chest.
    - **Infants:** Use two fingers to perform compressions, placing them just below the nipple line.

6. **Body Position:**
    - Keep your arms straight and use your upper body weight to perform compressions rather than relying solely on your arm strength.
    - Position your shoulders directly over your hands to apply adequate force.

7. **Compression Technique:**
    - Push down hard and fast, allowing the chest to return to its normal position between compressions.
    - Avoid leaning on the chest between compressions.

8. **Ventilations (if providing rescue breaths):**
    - Provide 2 rescue breaths after every 30 compressions (or 15 compressions if two rescuers are present for a child or infant).
    - Each breath should be given over 1 second and should cause visible chest rise.

Practical Tips for Effective Chest Compressions

1. **Check for Proper Compression Depth:**
    - Make sure you are pushing down to the correct depth. Compress the chest enough to make a noticeable indentation.
2. **Ensure Proper Hand Placement:**
    - Verify that your hands are correctly placed on the chest to avoid injury and to maximize compression effectiveness.

3. **Stay on Rhythm:**
    - Use a metronome or a rhythm-based device if available to maintain the correct compression rate. Otherwise, use the rhythm of a song like "Stayin' Alive" by the Bee Gees to keep pace.
4. **Use Full Body Weight:**
    - Engage your entire body weight to perform compressions rather than relying on just your arms.
5. **Monitor and Adjust:**
    - Periodically check to ensure compressions are effective and adjust as needed based on the patient's response and any changes in the situation.

Scenario Example: Performing High-Quality Chest Compressions

Scenario:

You are providing CPR to an adult who has collapsed and is unresponsive with no pulse.

Actions:

1. **Positioning:**
    - Place the patient on a firm, flat surface.
    - Kneel beside the patient and place the heel of one hand on the center of the chest, on the lower half of the sternum. Place your other hand on top and interlock your fingers.
2. **Perform Compressions:**
    - **Depth:** Push down at least 2 inches (5 cm) deep.
    - **Rate:** Compress the chest at a rate of 100-120 compressions per minute.
    - **Recoil:** Allow the chest to fully recoil between compressions.
3. **Continue CPR:**
    - Provide 30 compressions followed by 2 rescue breaths. Repeat the cycle continuously until emergency medical services arrive, the patient shows signs of life, or you are too exhausted to continue.

By consistently performing high-quality chest compressions, you maximize the chances of achieving a return of spontaneous circulation (ROSC) and improve the patient's chances of survival. Regular training and practice help to ensure that these skills are performed correctly and effectively.

Managing the airway effectively is essential in Basic Life Support (BLS) to ensure that oxygen can reach the lungs and prevent complications. Here's a step-by-step guide on how to manage the airway in BLS:

Steps to Manage the Airway in BLS

1. Check the Airway

- **Assess Responsiveness:**
  - Gently tap the patient and shout, "Are you okay?" to check if they are responsive.
- **Check Breathing:**
  - Look for chest rise and fall, listen for breath sounds, and feel for breath on your cheek. This should be done for no more than 10 seconds.

2. Open the Airway

- **Head-Tilt, Chin-Lift Maneuver (for unconscious patients):**
  - **Position the Patient:** Place the patient on their back on a firm, flat surface.
  - **Tilt the Head:** Place one hand on the patient's forehead and apply gentle pressure to tilt the head backward.
  - **Lift the Chin:** Use two fingers of your other hand to lift the chin upward, opening the airway. This maneuver helps lift the tongue off the back of the throat and opens the airway.
- **Jaw-Thrust Maneuver (if head or neck injury is suspected):**
  - **Position the Patient:** Place the patient on their back on a firm, flat surface.
  - **Thrust the Jaw:** Place your fingers behind the angle of the jaw and use your thumbs to push the lower jaw forward. This maneuver helps open the airway without tilting the head, which is important if a spinal injury is suspected.

3. Clear the Airway

- **Inspect the Mouth:**
    - **Check for Obstructions:** Look inside the patient's mouth for any visible obstructions such as food, vomit, or foreign objects.
    - **Remove Obstructions:** If you see an obstruction and it is easily reachable, use a finger sweep to remove it. Be careful not to push the object further down the throat.
- **Suctioning (if available):**
    - **Use Suction Device:** If you have access to a suction device, use it to clear the airway of secretions or fluids. Suction only as needed and avoid over-suctioning.

4. Provide Rescue Breaths

- **Use a Barrier Device (if available):**
    - **Place the Mask:** If you have a barrier device or pocket mask, place it over the patient's nose and mouth.
    - **Seal and Breathe:** Seal the mask against the patient's face and provide rescue breaths. Each breath should last about 1 second and should make the chest rise visibly.
- **Use Bag-Valve-Mask (BVM) (if trained and available):**
    - **Position the Mask:** Place the mask over the patient's nose and mouth and ensure a good seal.
    - **Bag Compression:** Squeeze the bag to provide breaths, each lasting about 1 second and ensuring visible chest rise.

5. Monitor and Reassess

- **Reassess the Airway:**
    - **Continue Monitoring:** Regularly check the patient's airway to ensure it remains open.
    - **Adjust as Needed:** If the patient's airway becomes obstructed again, reposition the head or use additional airway management techniques.
- **Ensure Effective Ventilation:**

- **Check Chest Rise:** Confirm that each rescue breath causes visible chest rise. This indicates that the breath is reaching the lungs.

6. Use Advanced Airway Devices (if trained):

- **Oropharyngeal Airway (OPA):**
  - **Measure and Insert:** Choose the correct size OPA and insert it with the curved side facing the roof of the mouth. Rotate it 180 degrees as it passes the tongue.
- **Nasopharyngeal Airway (NPA):**
  - **Measure and Insert:** Choose the appropriate size NPA and insert it gently into the nostril, lubricating it if needed.

Practical Tips for Airway Management

- **Maintain a Clear Airway:** Ensure that the airway remains clear of obstructions and is adequately opened.
- **Use Proper Techniques:** Use head-tilt, chin-lift or jaw-thrust maneuvers appropriately based on the patient's condition.
- **Check for Effectiveness:** Regularly assess if rescue breaths are effective by observing chest rise.
- **Avoid Overventilation:** Provide breaths at the recommended rate and volume to avoid complications from overventilation.

Scenario Example: Airway Management in Practice

Scenario:

You encounter an adult patient who is unresponsive and not breathing.

Actions:

1. **Position the Patient:**
   - Place the patient on their back on a firm, flat surface.
2. **Open the Airway:**
   - Use the head-tilt, chin-lift maneuver to open the airway.
3. **Clear the Airway:**

- Look inside the mouth for any visible obstructions and remove them if possible.
4. **Provide Rescue Breaths:**
    - Use a barrier device or BVM to provide rescue breaths, ensuring each breath causes visible chest rise.
5. **Monitor and Adjust:**
    - Continuously monitor the patient's airway and adjust your technique as needed.

By following these steps, you can effectively manage the airway and provide critical support to the patient until advanced medical help arrives. Regular practice and training in these techniques are essential for ensuring effective and timely care.

Trauma management in Basic Life Support (BLS) focuses on providing immediate care to individuals who have sustained injuries or trauma. The primary goals are to assess and manage life-threatening conditions, stabilize the patient, and prepare them for transport to advanced medical care. Here's a guide on how to manage trauma in BLS:

Trauma Management in BLS

1. Ensure Scene Safety

- **Assess the Scene:** Quickly evaluate the scene for any hazards or dangers (e.g., traffic, fire, chemical spills).
- **Protect Yourself and Others:** Ensure that the scene is safe for you and the patient. If necessary, move to a safer location.

2. Initial Assessment

- **Check Responsiveness:** Tap the patient and shout, "Are you okay?" to determine if they are responsive.
- **Call for Help:** If the patient is unresponsive or has a life-threatening injury, call for emergency medical services (EMS) immediately or send someone else to make the call.

3. Perform a Primary Survey (ABC)

- **Airway:**
  - **Open the Airway:** Use the head-tilt, chin-lift maneuver or jaw-thrust maneuver (if spinal injury is suspected) to open the airway.
  - **Check for Obstructions:** Look inside the mouth for obstructions and remove them if possible.
- **Breathing:**
  - **Assess Breathing:** Look for chest rise and fall, listen for breath sounds, and feel for breath on your cheek.
  - **Provide Rescue Breaths:** If the patient is not breathing, give rescue breaths using a barrier device or bag-valve-mask (BVM).
- **Circulation:**
  - **Check Pulse:** Assess for a pulse at the carotid (adults) or brachial (infants) pulse point.
  - **Control Severe Bleeding:** Look for severe external bleeding. Apply direct pressure to wounds to control bleeding.

4. Perform a Secondary Survey

- **Examine the Patient:**
  - **Head-to-Toe Assessment:** Check for additional injuries, including deformities, bruising, or tenderness.
  - **Assess Vital Signs:** Monitor heart rate, blood pressure, and respiratory rate if possible.
- **Look for Specific Injuries:**
  - **Head and Neck:** Check for signs of head trauma or spinal injury.
  - **Chest:** Look for signs of rib fractures, pneumothorax, or other chest injuries.
  - **Abdomen:** Assess for signs of abdominal injury, such as distention or tenderness.
  - **Pelvis and Extremities:** Check for possible fractures or dislocations.

5. Manage Specific Trauma Situations

- **Spinal Injury:**

- **Immobilize the Spine:** Keep the patient's head and neck in a neutral position. Avoid moving the patient unless absolutely necessary.
- **Use a Cervical Collar:** If available, apply a cervical collar to help stabilize the neck.
- Fractures and Dislocations:
    - **Immobilize Injuries:** Use splints or improvised materials to immobilize fractured or dislocated limbs. Avoid moving the patient's limb unless it is causing further injury.
- Chest Injuries:
    - **Flail Chest:** Stabilize flail segments with a dressing or support. Encourage the patient to breathe deeply.
    - **Pneumothorax:** Apply an occlusive dressing to any open chest wounds to prevent air from entering the chest cavity.
- Abdominal Injuries:
    - **Cover Open Wounds:** Use a sterile dressing or clean cloth to cover open abdominal wounds. Do not attempt to push any protruding organs back inside.

6. Prepare for Transport

- Stabilize the Patient:
    - **Ensure Comfort:** Make sure the patient is as comfortable as possible and continue monitoring vital signs.
    - **Minimize Movement:** Avoid unnecessary movement, especially if spinal injury is suspected.
- Communicate with EMS:
    - **Provide Information:** Give emergency responders a clear report of the patient's condition, including any trauma injuries, interventions performed, and the patient's response to treatment.

7. Continuous Monitoring and Reassessment

- **Reassess the Patient:** Continuously monitor the patient's condition and adjust your care as needed.
- **Watch for Changes:** Be alert for any changes in the patient's status, such as worsening of injuries or signs of shock.

Practical Tips for Trauma Management

- **Use Appropriate PPE:** Wear personal protective equipment, such as gloves and masks, to protect yourself and the patient.
- **Be Efficient and Calm:** Perform assessments and interventions efficiently while maintaining a calm demeanor to reduce stress for both you and the patient.
- **Work with a Team:** If possible, work with other rescuers to divide tasks and provide effective care.

Scenario Example: Trauma Management in Practice

Scenario:

You arrive at the scene of a car accident and find an adult patient who is unresponsive and has visible external bleeding.

Actions:

1. **Ensure Scene Safety:** Make sure the scene is safe for you and the patient.
2. **Initial Assessment:**
    - Check for responsiveness and call for help.
    - Open the airway using the head-tilt, chin-lift maneuver.
    - Assess breathing and pulse. Provide rescue breaths if needed.
3. **Control Bleeding:**
    - Apply direct pressure to the wound to control severe bleeding.
4. **Secondary Survey:**
    - Perform a head-to-toe assessment to identify other injuries.
5. **Manage Specific Injuries:**
    - If spinal injury is suspected, immobilize the spine and apply a cervical collar if available.
    - Immobilize any fractured limbs using splints.
6. **Prepare for Transport:**
    - Stabilize the patient and minimize movement.
    - Communicate with EMS and provide a detailed report.
7. **Continuous Monitoring:**

- Regularly reassess the patient and adjust care as needed.

By following these steps, you can provide effective trauma management in BLS, stabilize the patient, and improve their chances of a favorable outcome. Regular training and practice are essential for maintaining these skills.

Treating burns effectively in Basic Life Support (BLS) involves managing the injury to minimize damage, prevent complications, and provide comfort until advanced medical care is available. Here's a guide on how to treat burns in BLS:

Steps to Treat Burns in BLS

1. Ensure Scene Safety

- **Assess the Scene:** Ensure that the environment is safe before approaching the patient. Remove any potential hazards or dangers, such as flames or electrical sources.

2. Initial Assessment

- **Check Responsiveness:** Determine if the patient is responsive and assess their condition. Check their airway, breathing, and circulation (ABCs).
- **Call for Help:** If the burn is severe or if the patient is unresponsive, call for emergency medical services (EMS) or send someone else to make the call.

3. Manage the Burn Injury

- **Stop the Burning Process:**
  - **Remove the Patient from Danger:** If the patient is still in contact with the source of the burn (e.g., flames or electricity), move them to a safe location if it is safe to do so.
  - **Extinguish Flames:** If the patient's clothing is on fire, use a fire blanket or a heavy cloth to extinguish the flames. Do not use water if the patient is involved in a chemical burn scenario.

- **Cool the Burn:**
  - **Apply Cool Water:** Use cool (not cold) running water to gently cool the burn area. Do this for at least 10 minutes to help reduce pain and prevent further tissue damage.
  - **Avoid Ice:** Do not apply ice directly to the burn as it can cause further damage to the tissue.
- **Protect the Burn:**
  - **Cover the Burn:** Use a clean, non-stick dressing or cloth to cover the burn. If possible, use a sterile dressing to reduce the risk of infection.
  - **Avoid Applying Ointments or Creams:** Do not apply ointments, creams, or home remedies to the burn as they may cause infection or interfere with medical treatment.

4. Assess the Severity of the Burn

- **Determine Burn Depth:**
  - **First-Degree Burns:** Affect only the outer layer of the skin (epidermis) and cause redness, mild swelling, and pain.
  - **Second-Degree Burns:** Affect both the outer layer and the underlying layer of skin (dermis), causing redness, swelling, blistering, and pain.
  - **Third-Degree Burns:** Extend through all layers of the skin and may involve deeper tissues. The skin may appear white, charred, or leathery, and there may be no pain due to nerve damage.
- **Assess the Burn Area:**
  - **Calculate the Burn Area:** Use the "Rule of Nines" to estimate the total body surface area (TBSA) affected by the burn. For adults, the body is divided into sections (e.g., head and neck = 9%, each arm = 9%, each leg = 18%, etc.).
  - **Consider Special Areas:** Burns on the face, hands, feet, or genitals, or those that cover large areas, require special attention.

5. Monitor and Provide Comfort

- **Monitor for Shock:**

- **Check Vital Signs:** Monitor the patient's pulse, breathing, and level of consciousness.
- **Look for Signs of Shock:** Symptoms may include pale skin, rapid breathing, weakness, or confusion. If shock is suspected, keep the patient warm and comfortable.
- Provide Comfort:
  - **Reassure the Patient:** Offer reassurance and keep them calm. Pain management is important; however, avoid giving the patient anything to eat or drink if advanced medical care is imminent.

6. Prepare for Transport

- Stabilize the Patient:
  - **Continue Cooling and Covering:** Maintain cooling of the burn and ensure that the burn is covered with a clean, dry dressing.
  - **Avoid Unnecessary Movement:** Minimize movement of the burned area to prevent further injury.
- Communicate with EMS:
  - **Provide Detailed Information:** Inform emergency responders about the burn's location, extent, and any treatments provided.

Practical Tips for Burn Management

- **Avoid Direct Contact with Burned Skin:** Use clean materials to handle the burn and avoid direct contact with the burned area.
- **Be Cautious with Chemicals:** For chemical burns, ensure that any chemicals are removed from the skin and follow specific protocols for the type of chemical involved.
- **Keep the Patient Hydrated:** If the patient is conscious and able to drink, offer small sips of water to help with hydration.

Scenario Example: Treating a Burn in Practice

Scenario:

You encounter a patient who has sustained a second-degree burn to the arm from a hot liquid.

Actions:

1. **Ensure Scene Safety:** Confirm that the environment is safe and there are no ongoing hazards.
2. **Initial Assessment:**
    - Check the patient's responsiveness and call for help if needed.
    - Open the airway, assess breathing, and check for a pulse.
3. **Manage the Burn:**
    - **Cool the Burn:** Gently apply cool running water to the burn area for at least 10 minutes.
    - **Protect the Burn:** Cover the burn with a clean, non-stick dressing.
4. **Assess the Burn Severity:**
    - Recognize the second-degree burn with blistering and pain.
5. **Monitor and Comfort:**
    - Monitor the patient for signs of shock and provide comfort.
6. **Prepare for Transport:**
    - Stabilize the patient and communicate details to EMS.

By following these steps, you can effectively manage burn injuries in BLS, reducing damage and providing essential care until advanced medical treatment is available. Regular training and practice help to ensure these skills are performed accurately and efficiently.

Helping with a birth in Basic Life Support (BLS) involves providing assistance in a safe and supportive manner until advanced medical care arrives. While BLS guidelines don't cover the full scope of childbirth, you can offer critical support during a delivery by following these steps:

Steps to Assist with Childbirth in BLS

1. Ensure Scene Safety

- **Assess the Scene:** Ensure that the environment is safe and free of hazards. Ensure privacy and comfort for the mother.

2. Call for Help

- **Activate Emergency Services:** Call for emergency medical services (EMS) immediately if you suspect complications or if you are unsure of the situation.
- **Provide Information:** Give clear details about the situation, including the mother's condition, expected delivery, and any complications.

3. Prepare for Delivery

- **Wash Hands:** If possible, wash your hands or use hand sanitizer to ensure cleanliness.
- **Prepare Materials:** Gather clean towels, blankets, or cloths. If available, use sterile gloves.

4. Assist with Delivery

- **Support the Mother:**
  - **Help the Mother to a Comfortable Position:** If the mother is able, encourage her to lie on her back with knees bent or to adopt a position that is comfortable for her.
  - **Encourage Breathing and Pushing:** Support the mother with breathing techniques and encourage her to push during contractions.
- **Assist with Delivery:**
  - **Support the Baby's Head:** As the baby's head emerges, use clean towels to support and gently guide it. Do not pull on the baby.
  - **Avoid Pressing on the Abdomen:** Do not apply pressure to the abdomen or attempt to deliver the baby unless it is necessary and you are trained to do so.
- **Deliver the Baby:**
  - **Guide the Baby Out:** Gently guide the baby's head and shoulders out, allowing the body to follow. Support the baby as it is delivered.

- **Clear the Airway:** Once the baby is born, gently clear any mucus or fluids from the baby's mouth and nose with a bulb syringe if available.

5. Care for the Baby

- **Stimulate Breathing:** If the baby is not crying or breathing, gently stimulate the baby by rubbing the back or tapping the feet.
- **Warm the Baby:** Place the baby on a clean, dry towel and wrap them to keep warm. Ensure that the baby is in a safe, warm environment.

6. Care for the Mother

- **Help with the Placenta:** Once the baby is delivered, help the mother with the delivery of the placenta. Encourage her to push as needed, but do not pull on the placenta.
- **Monitor for Complications:** Watch for any signs of excessive bleeding, shock, or complications. Support the mother and keep her calm.
- **Comfort and Reassure:** Offer emotional support to the mother. Reassure her that help is on the way and keep her as comfortable as possible.

7. Prepare for Transport

- **Stabilize the Mother and Baby:** Ensure both the mother and baby are stable and comfortable.
- **Provide Information to EMS:** When EMS arrives, provide a clear report of the delivery, including any complications and the condition of both the mother and baby.

Practical Tips for Assisting with Childbirth

- **Stay Calm and Supportive:** Provide reassurance to the mother and remain calm throughout the process.
- **Respect Privacy:** Ensure that the environment is as private and comfortable as possible.

- **Follow Basic Protocols:** Use clean materials and avoid introducing any unnecessary risks.

Scenario Example: Assisting with Childbirth

Scenario:

You arrive at the scene and find a woman in labor with visible contractions.

Actions:

1. **Ensure Scene Safety:** Confirm that the environment is safe and private.
2. **Call for Help:** Activate emergency services and provide details about the situation.
3. **Prepare for Delivery:**
    - Wash your hands and gather clean towels.
4. **Assist with Delivery:**
    - Help the mother to a comfortable position and encourage her to push.
    - Support the baby's head as it emerges and guide the baby out gently.
5. **Care for the Baby:**
    - Clear the baby's airway and stimulate breathing if necessary.
    - Wrap the baby to keep warm.
6. **Care for the Mother:**
    - Assist with the delivery of the placenta and monitor for complications.
    - Offer comfort and reassurance.
7. **Prepare for Transport:**
    - Ensure both the mother and baby are stable and provide a detailed report to EMS.

By following these steps, you can provide crucial support during a childbirth situation and ensure that both the mother and baby receive appropriate care until advanced medical professionals arrive.

Treating a knife injury in a basic life support (BLS) situation involves several critical steps. Here's a general approach:

1. **Ensure Safety**: Make sure the scene is safe for you and the injured person. If necessary, call for emergency medical services (EMS) before providing any assistance.
2. **Assess the Situation**: Check the person's responsiveness and breathing. If they are unconscious and not breathing, start CPR. If they are conscious, continue with the following steps.
3. **Control Bleeding**:
    - **Apply Direct Pressure**: Use a clean cloth or bandage and apply firm, direct pressure to the wound to control bleeding. If the cloth becomes soaked, do not remove it; add more layers on top.
    - **Keep the Person Calm**: Encourage them to remain as still and calm as possible to reduce bleeding.
4. **Protect the Wound**:
    - If the knife is still embedded in the wound, do not remove it. Instead, stabilize the knife by gently holding it in place with clean cloths or bandages to prevent movement and further bleeding.
    - If the knife is removed, cover the wound with a clean bandage or cloth and apply pressure.
5. **Monitor for Shock**: Watch for signs of shock, such as pale or clammy skin, rapid breathing, or confusion. If these symptoms are present, lay the person down with their legs elevated (if possible) and keep them warm with a blanket.
6. **Do Not Use Tourniquets**: Unless you're specifically trained to use them and there's severe limb bleeding, avoid using tourniquets as they can cause further harm.
7. **Seek Medical Attention**: Ensure that the person gets professional medical help as soon as possible, even if the wound appears minor.
8. **Provide Reassurance**: Keep the person as calm and reassured as possible while waiting for professional help.

Remember, this advice is for immediate response and should not replace professional medical treatment.

Managing fractures and dislocations in a Basic Life Support (BLS) situation involves several key steps to stabilize the injury and prevent further harm. Here's how to handle each type:

Fractures

1. **Assess the Injury:**
   - Check for signs of a fracture, such as pain, swelling, bruising, or deformity.
2. **Immobilize the Fracture:**
   - **Do Not Move the Injured Person**: If possible, avoid moving the injured person to prevent further injury.
   - **Immobilize the Limb**: Use a splint or any rigid material (e.g., a board, rolled-up magazine) to keep the broken bone in place. Immobilize both the joints above and below the fracture site.
   - **Padding**: Place padding (e.g., cloth) between the splint and the skin to reduce pressure and friction.
3. **Apply Ice:**
   - If available, apply ice packs wrapped in cloth to the area to reduce swelling and pain. Avoid placing ice directly on the skin.
4. **Monitor for Shock:**
   - Watch for signs of shock, such as pale or clammy skin, rapid breathing, or confusion. Keep the person warm and calm.
5. **Seek Medical Help:**
   - Ensure that the person receives professional medical evaluation and treatment as soon as possible.

Dislocations

1. **Assess the Injury:**
   - Look for symptoms like intense pain, visible deformity, or inability to move the joint.
2. **Immobilize the Joint:**
   - **Do Not Attempt to Relocate**: Do not try to reposition the dislocated joint yourself. This can cause further damage.

- **Support the Joint**: Use a sling or another method to support and immobilize the joint in its current position.
3. **Apply Ice**:
    - Apply ice packs wrapped in cloth to the area to reduce pain and swelling.
4. **Monitor for Shock**:
    - Similar to fractures, be attentive to signs of shock and manage accordingly.
5. **Seek Medical Help**:
    - Prompt professional medical attention is essential to properly relocate the joint and assess any associated damage.

In both cases, communication with emergency services is crucial. Inform them of the injuries and your management actions so they can provide appropriate care upon arrival.

Managing head, neck, and spine injuries in Basic Life Support (BLS) situations requires careful handling to prevent further injury. Here's a step-by-step guide:

Head Injuries

1. **Assess the Situation**:
    - Check for responsiveness and signs of a serious injury such as loss of consciousness, confusion, or severe headache.
2. **Immobilize the Head**:
    - If the person is unconscious or suspected to have a head injury, avoid moving them. Stabilize the head and neck to prevent further movement.
3. **Monitor and Provide Support**:
    - Observe for signs of a concussion or more severe brain injury, such as vomiting, seizures, or irregular breathing.
    - Keep the person comfortable and calm, but avoid giving food or drink.
4. **Seek Medical Help**:
    - Immediate medical evaluation is essential for head injuries, especially if there is loss of consciousness or worsening symptoms.

Neck Injuries

1. **Assess the Situation:**
   - Look for signs of neck pain, limited movement, or neurological symptoms (e.g., numbness, tingling, or weakness).
2. **Immobilize the Neck:**
   - Keep the person's head and neck as still as possible. Use your hands or a makeshift cervical collar if available to stabilize the neck.
   - Avoid any movement of the person, and do not try to reposition them.
3. **Monitor and Provide Support:**
   - Watch for symptoms of shock or respiratory difficulties and manage them accordingly.
   - Do not attempt to manipulate or realign the neck.
4. **Seek Medical Help:**
   - Immediate professional medical evaluation is crucial for neck injuries to prevent complications.

Spine Injuries

1. **Assess the Situation:**
   - Look for signs of spinal injury, such as pain along the spine, difficulty moving, or changes in sensation or strength.
2. **Immobilize the Spine:**
   - Keep the person as still as possible. If they are lying on their back, ensure their body is aligned in a neutral position.
   - Do not move the person unless necessary to prevent further danger (e.g., from a hazardous environment).
3. **Support the Head and Neck:**
   - Use supports or rolled-up towels to stabilize the head and neck if they are not already immobilized.
4. **Monitor and Provide Support:**
   - Watch for changes in their condition and be prepared to manage shock or respiratory issues if they arise.
5. **Seek Medical Help:**

- Immediate medical attention is necessary for suspected spinal injuries to ensure proper treatment and prevent long-term damage.

In all cases, avoid any unnecessary movement of the injured person to minimize the risk of aggravating the injury. Providing accurate information to emergency responders will help them deliver appropriate care.

Managing chest injuries in Basic Life Support (BLS) involves careful assessment and intervention to prevent complications. Here's a step-by-step approach:

1. Assess the Injury

- **Check for Breathing**: Determine if the person is breathing normally. Look for signs of difficulty breathing, such as rapid or shallow breathing, or any use of accessory muscles.
- **Look for Symptoms**: Signs may include severe pain in the chest, difficulty breathing, cyanosis (bluish discoloration of the skin), or abnormal chest movement.

2. Stabilize the Person

- **Positioning**: If the person is conscious, have them sit up or lean forward slightly to ease breathing. If they are unconscious or unable to sit up, place them in a recovery position or with the head elevated if it helps with breathing.

3. Manage Specific Types of Chest Injuries

- **Flail Chest:**
  - **Immobilize the Flail Segment**: Apply gentle pressure to the flail segment (the part of the chest that moves independently) to stabilize it. This can be done using a bulky dressing or hand if no other material is available.
  - **Monitor Breathing**: Ensure that the person continues to breathe and be prepared to provide support as needed.
- **Punctured Lung (Sucking Chest Wound):**

- **Seal the Wound:** If there is an open wound causing air to be sucked in and out of the chest, cover it with a sterile dressing or plastic wrap. Tape it down on three sides, leaving one side open to allow air to escape but not enter. This helps prevent a buildup of air in the chest cavity (tension pneumothorax).
    - **Monitor for Changes:** Watch for worsening symptoms and changes in breathing or consciousness.
- **Blunt Trauma:**
    - **Apply Ice:** If available, apply ice wrapped in a cloth to the injured area to reduce pain and swelling.
    - **Monitor for Internal Injuries:** Watch for signs of more severe internal injury, such as difficulty breathing or a drop in blood pressure.

4. Monitor and Manage Shock

- **Watch for Shock:** Signs include pale or clammy skin, rapid pulse, or confusion. Manage shock by keeping the person warm, lying down with their legs elevated (if not contraindicated by injury), and reassuring them.
- **Provide Oxygen:** If available and trained, provide supplemental oxygen to assist with breathing.

5. Seek Medical Help

- **Call for Emergency Services:** Ensure that the person receives professional medical evaluation and treatment as soon as possible. Provide details about the injury and your management actions.

6. Document and Communicate

- **Record Observations:** Document any symptoms, changes in the person's condition, and the care provided.
- **Communicate Clearly:** When emergency services arrive, clearly communicate what you have observed and the steps you have taken.

Proper management of chest injuries can significantly affect the outcome, so maintaining stability and minimizing movement are key to preventing further harm.

Managing abdominal injuries in Basic Life Support (BLS) involves steps to stabilize the injury and prevent further complications. Here's a guide for handling such injuries:

1. Assess the Injury

- **Check for Symptoms**: Look for signs such as severe abdominal pain, swelling, bruising, or any visible wounds. The person may also have nausea, vomiting, or signs of shock.
- **Determine Consciousness**: Ensure the person is conscious and responsive. If unconscious, check for breathing and pulse.

2. Manage External Wounds

- **Cover the Wound**: If there is an open wound or evisceration (internal organs protruding), cover the area with a sterile dressing or clean cloth.
    - **Do Not Push Protruding Organs Back**: If organs are protruding, do not attempt to push them back into the abdomen. Instead, cover them with a moist (not soaking wet) sterile dressing or cloth to keep them moist and protected.
- **Apply Gentle Pressure**: If there is bleeding, apply gentle pressure around the wound to control it. Avoid applying too much pressure which could worsen the injury.

3. Position the Person

- **Comfortable Position**: Have the person lie on their back with their knees bent if it is comfortable for them. This position can help reduce abdominal pain by relaxing the abdominal muscles.
- **Avoid Movement**: Minimize movement to avoid aggravating the injury.

4. Monitor and Manage Shock

- **Watch for Signs of Shock**: Symptoms include pale, cool, or clammy skin, rapid pulse, shallow breathing, or confusion.
  - **Keep the Person Warm**: Cover them with a blanket or clothing to maintain body temperature.
  - **Elevate Legs**: If not contraindicated by other injuries, elevate the person's legs slightly to improve blood flow to vital organs.

5. Provide Support

- **Reassure the Person**: Keep them calm and reassured while waiting for emergency services.
- **Do Not Give Food or Drink**: Avoid giving the person food or drink, as this may complicate surgery or treatment.

6. Seek Medical Help

- **Call Emergency Services**: Ensure professional medical evaluation and treatment are on the way. Provide details about the injury and the care you've administered.

7. Document and Communicate

- **Record Observations**: Document the person's symptoms, changes in their condition, and the care you provided.
- **Communicate Clearly**: When emergency responders arrive, clearly explain the injury and the steps taken to manage it.

Important Notes

- **Avoid Direct Pressure on Severe Injuries**: For severe abdominal injuries with suspected internal damage, avoid applying direct pressure to prevent further harm.
- **Handle with Care**: Always handle the person gently to avoid causing additional pain or damage.

Prompt and appropriate management of abdominal injuries can significantly impact the outcome, so maintaining stability and minimizing further injury are crucial.

Treating an eye injury in Basic Life Support (BLS) requires careful handling to prevent further damage and alleviate discomfort. Here's how to manage eye injuries:

1. Assess the Injury

- **Check for Symptoms**: Look for signs such as redness, swelling, pain, blurred vision, or foreign objects in the eye. Ask the person about their symptoms and any potential causes of the injury.

2. Manage Foreign Objects

- **Do Not Rub the Eye**: Advise the person to avoid rubbing the eye, as this can worsen the injury.
- **Flush the Eye**: If a small foreign object (e.g., dust, sand) is in the eye and not embedded, gently flush the eye with clean water or saline solution. Use an eyewash station if available, or pour water gently from a clean container.
- **Remove Visible Objects**: If the object is on the surface of the eye and easily visible, use a clean cloth or sterile pad to carefully remove it. Avoid using sharp objects or tweezers.

3. Manage Chemical Burns

- **Irrigate the Eye**: Rinse the eye with copious amounts of clean water or saline solution immediately. Rinse for at least 15-20 minutes, making sure the water flows from the inner corner of the eye to the outer corner to avoid washing chemicals into the other eye.
- **Remove Contact Lenses**: If the person is wearing contact lenses, remove them as soon as possible during irrigation.

4. Manage Trauma

- **Protect the Eye**: If there is significant trauma, cover the eye with a sterile dressing or clean cloth. Avoid putting pressure on the eye.
- **Do Not Apply Pressure**: Avoid applying pressure to the injured eye, especially if there is a risk of penetration or rupture.

5. Monitor for Symptoms

- **Check Vision**: Assess if there is any change in vision. If vision is significantly impaired or if there is severe pain, these could indicate more serious injuries.
- **Watch for Signs of Infection**: Look for redness, increased pain, or discharge, which may indicate an infection.

6. Seek Medical Help

- **Call for Professional Medical Assistance**: Ensure the person gets evaluated by a medical professional as soon as possible. Eye injuries can range from minor to severe, and timely intervention is crucial.

7. Provide Support

- **Reassure the Person**: Keep the person calm and reassure them while waiting for emergency services.
- **Avoid Food or Drink**: Do not give the person food or drink until a medical professional has assessed them.

8. Document and Communicate

- **Record Observations**: Note any symptoms, changes in the condition, and the steps you took to manage the injury.
- **Communicate Clearly**: Provide emergency responders with clear information about the injury and the care administered.

Important Notes

- **Avoid Putting Anything in the Eye**: Do not use any ointments or medications without medical advice.
- **Handle with Care**: Be gentle to avoid causing additional pain or harm.

Proper management of eye injuries can prevent complications and aid in a faster recovery.

In Basic Life Support (BLS), recognizing and managing different types of shock is crucial for providing appropriate care. Shock is a medical emergency that occurs when the body's organs and tissues do not receive enough blood flow. Here are the main types of shock you might encounter:

1. Hypovolemic Shock

Cause: Severe loss of blood or fluids from the body, often due to trauma, internal bleeding, or dehydration.

Signs and Symptoms:

- Rapid, weak pulse
- Low blood pressure
- Pale, cool, or clammy skin
- Rapid, shallow breathing
- Thirst
- Confusion or lethargy

Management:

- **Control Bleeding**: Apply direct pressure to any visible bleeding wounds.
- **Position the Person**: Lay them flat and elevate their legs (unless contraindicated by injuries).
- **Maintain Body Temperature**: Keep them warm with a blanket.
- **Seek Medical Help**: Ensure professional medical assistance is on the way.

2. Cardiogenic Shock

Cause: The heart is unable to pump effectively due to conditions like heart attack or severe heart failure.

Signs and Symptoms:

- Weak or rapid pulse
- Low blood pressure
- Shortness of breath

- Cyanosis (bluish skin, especially around the lips or fingers)
- Chest pain
- Confusion or altered mental status

Management:

- **Comfort the Person**: Have them sit up or lie in a comfortable position if they are having difficulty breathing.
- **Monitor Vital Signs**: Keep track of their pulse, breathing, and level of consciousness.
- **Seek Medical Help**: Immediate professional medical attention is essential.

3. Distributive Shock

Types: Includes septic shock, anaphylactic shock, and neurogenic shock.

- Septic Shock:
    - **Cause**: Severe infection leading to systemic inflammation and blood vessel dilation.
    - **Signs**: Fever, chills, rapid breathing, confusion, and low blood pressure.
    - **Management**: Provide comfort, monitor vital signs, and seek immediate medical attention.
- Anaphylactic Shock:
    - **Cause**: Severe allergic reaction causing widespread vasodilation and airway constriction.
    - **Signs**: Difficulty breathing, hives, swelling, low blood pressure, rapid pulse.
    - **Management**: If available, administer epinephrine (if trained). Support breathing and seek emergency medical help immediately.
- Neurogenic Shock:
    - **Cause**: Severe damage to the spinal cord or nervous system leading to blood vessel dilation.
    - **Signs**: Low blood pressure, warm and dry skin, slow heart rate.

- **Management**: Stabilize the person's position, monitor vital signs, and ensure prompt medical assistance.

4. Obstructive Shock

Cause: Physical obstruction in the circulation, such as from a pulmonary embolism or cardiac tamponade.

Signs and Symptoms:

- Difficulty breathing
- Sharp chest pain
- Rapid heart rate
- Low blood pressure
- Cyanosis

Management:

- **Comfort the Person**: Position them to ease breathing if necessary.
- **Monitor Vital Signs**: Watch for changes and be prepared to perform CPR if needed.
- **Seek Immediate Medical Help**: Professional intervention is crucial to address the underlying cause.

General Management for Shock

1. **Assess and Monitor**: Continuously monitor vital signs (pulse, breathing, blood pressure) and level of consciousness.
2. **Position the Person**: Generally, lay them flat with legs elevated unless there are contraindications.
3. **Maintain Warmth**: Keep the person warm with a blanket or clothing.
4. **Provide Reassurance**: Keep the person calm and reassure them while waiting for professional medical help.

Recognizing and managing shock promptly can significantly improve outcomes and reduce the risk of complications.

In Basic Life Support (BLS), various types of medical equipment are used to provide immediate care and stabilize patients. Here's an overview of commonly used equipment:

1. Automated External Defibrillator (AED)

- **Purpose**: Provides electric shocks to restore a normal heart rhythm in cases of cardiac arrest.
- **Usage**: Place electrode pads on the patient's chest as directed by the AED. Follow the device's voice and visual prompts.

2. Bag-Valve-Mask (BVM)

- **Purpose**: Assists with breathing by delivering positive pressure ventilation.
- **Usage**: Seal the mask over the patient's nose and mouth, squeeze the bag to deliver breaths, and ensure proper ventilation.

3. Oxygen Equipment

- **Purpose**: Provides supplemental oxygen to patients with respiratory distress or low oxygen levels.
- **Components**:
    - **Oxygen Cylinder**: Portable tank containing oxygen.
    - **Oxygen Regulator**: Controls the flow rate of oxygen.
    - **Oxygen Mask or Cannula**: Delivers oxygen to the patient's airway.

4. Suction Device

- **Purpose**: Clears the airway of secretions, blood, or other obstructions.
- **Usage**: Use suction tubing and a catheter to remove obstructions from the patient's airway.

5. Pulse Oximeter

- **Purpose**: Measures oxygen saturation levels in the blood.
- **Usage**: Attach the device to the patient's finger, toe, or earlobe to obtain a reading of blood oxygen levels.

6. Blood Pressure Cuff and Stethoscope

- **Purpose**: Measures blood pressure.
- **Usage**: Place the cuff around the patient's upper arm, inflate it, and use the stethoscope to listen for Korotkoff sounds to determine blood pressure readings.

7. Trauma Dressings and Bandages

- **Purpose**: Control bleeding and protect wounds.
- **Components**:
    - **Sterile Dressings**: Cover and protect wounds.
    - **Bandages**: Secure dressings and immobilize injuries.
    - **Trauma Kits**: Often include large, absorbent dressings for heavy bleeding.

8. Splints

- **Purpose**: Immobilize and stabilize fractures or dislocations.
- **Types**:
    - **Rigid Splints**: Made from materials like plastic or metal.
    - **Soft Splints**: Made from foam or other pliable materials.

9. Cervical Collar

- **Purpose**: Stabilizes and immobilizes the neck to prevent spinal injury.
- **Usage**: Apply around the patient's neck to keep it aligned and immobilized.

10. Glucometer

- **Purpose**: Measures blood glucose levels.
- **Usage**: Use a lancet to obtain a small blood sample and place it on a test strip to measure glucose levels.

11. Emergency Blankets

- **Purpose**: Provides warmth and helps maintain body temperature.

- **Usage:** Cover the patient to prevent hypothermia and maintain comfort.

12. Personal Protective Equipment (PPE)

- **Purpose:** Protects the rescuer from exposure to bodily fluids or infectious agents.
- **Components:**
    - **Gloves:** Protect hands during patient care.
    - **Masks and Eye Protection:** Protect from airborne particles or splashes.
    - **Gowns:** Provide additional protection during patient care.

13. Airway Management Tools

- **Purpose:** Ensure a clear and open airway.
- **Types:**
    - **Oropharyngeal Airways (OPA):** Keeps the airway open by preventing the tongue from blocking it.
    - **Nasopharyngeal Airways (NPA):** An alternative to OPA, used when the patient has a gag reflex.

These tools are integral to performing effective BLS and providing critical care in emergency situations. Proper use and knowledge of this equipment are essential for successful patient management and stabilization.

Using an Automated External Defibrillator (AED) is a critical component of Basic Life Support (BLS) when dealing with a person experiencing cardiac arrest. Here's a step-by-step guide on how to use an AED:

1. Ensure Safety

- **Check the Scene:** Ensure the environment is safe for both you and the patient.
- **Confirm Unresponsiveness:** Gently shake the person and shout to see if they respond. If unresponsive, proceed with the AED.

2. Call for Help

- **Activate Emergency Services**: Call for emergency medical assistance immediately or direct someone else to do so.
- **Get the AED**: If not already on-site, have someone bring the AED.

3. Prepare the Person

- **Place the Person on a Firm Surface**: Ensure the patient is on a hard, flat surface (e.g., the floor).
- **Expose the Chest**: Remove or cut away clothing from the chest to expose bare skin. Dry the chest if it's wet or sweaty.

4. Apply AED Pads

- **Open the AED**: Turn on the AED by pressing the power button. Follow the voice and visual prompts.
- **Apply the Pads**: Place the electrode pads on the patient's chest as follows:
    - **Adult Pads**: One pad on the upper right chest (above the nipple) and the other pad on the lower left side of the chest (below the armpit).
    - **Child Pads**: Follow specific instructions for pad placement if using pediatric pads.

5. Connect the Pads

- **Attach the Pads**: Connect the electrode pads to the AED machine if they are not pre-connected.
- **Ensure Good Contact**: Press the pads firmly onto the chest to ensure good contact with the skin.

6. Analyze the Heart Rhythm

- **Stand Clear**: Ensure no one is touching the patient.
- **Press the Analyze Button**: The AED will automatically analyze the heart rhythm to determine if a shock is needed. Do not touch the patient during this time.

7. Deliver a Shock

- **Follow Prompts:** If the AED advises a shock, ensure everyone is clear of the patient.
- **Press the Shock Button:** Deliver the shock by pressing the indicated button. Ensure that no one is in contact with the patient during the shock.

8. Continue Care

- **Resume CPR:** After delivering the shock, immediately resume chest compressions and rescue breaths (if trained and able) as per BLS guidelines.
- **Follow AED Prompts:** The AED will provide further instructions and may re-analyze the rhythm after a few minutes.
- **Reapply Pads if Needed:** If the AED indicates a shock is needed again, ensure the pads remain properly placed and deliver another shock if advised.

9. Post-Event Care

- **Monitor the Patient:** Continue to monitor the patient's condition until emergency services arrive.
- **Provide Information:** When emergency responders arrive, provide them with details about the patient's condition and the care provided.

Important Considerations

- **Pediatric Use:** Use pediatric pads and settings for children under 8 years old or less than 55 pounds, if available. Follow specific guidelines for pediatric AED use.
- **Battery and Maintenance:** Ensure the AED's battery is charged and that the device is properly maintained and ready for use.

Using an AED correctly can significantly improve the chances of survival in cases of cardiac arrest. Following these steps ensures that you provide effective and timely assistance.

Using a Bag-Valve-Mask (BVM) in Basic Life Support (BLS) is a crucial skill for providing effective positive pressure ventilation to patients who are not breathing adequately. Here's a step-by-step guide on how to use a BVM:

1. Ensure Safety and Check Responsiveness

- **Check the Scene**: Ensure that the environment is safe for both you and the patient.
- **Confirm Unresponsiveness**: Gently shake the person and shout to see if they respond. If unresponsive and not breathing or breathing inadequately, proceed with BVM ventilation.

2. Open the Airway

- **Use the Head-Tilt, Chin-Lift**: If the patient is lying on their back, tilt their head back and lift the chin to open the airway. Alternatively, use the Jaw-Thrust maneuver if there is suspected spinal injury.
- **Ensure Airway is Clear**: Check for any obstructions and remove them if necessary.

3. Prepare the BVM Equipment

- **Assemble the BVM**: Ensure that the BVM unit includes a bag, valve, and mask. Check that the mask is clean and the bag is functioning properly.
- **Connect the Oxygen (if available)**: Attach the oxygen tubing to the BVM and turn on the oxygen flow if you have access to supplemental oxygen.

4. Position the Mask

- **Select the Appropriate Mask Size**: Choose a mask that fits the patient's face properly.
- **Seal the Mask**: Place the mask over the patient's nose and mouth, ensuring a good seal. The mask should cover both the nose and mouth.

5. Use the BVM

- **Seal the Mask**: Using both hands, create an airtight seal around the mask by pressing it firmly against the patient's face.
    - **C-E Grip**: Use your thumb and index finger to form a "C" shape on the top of the mask, while your other fingers form an "E" shape on the jaw to stabilize the mask and hold the airway open.
- **Squeeze the Bag**: With your other hand, squeeze the bag to deliver breaths. Each squeeze should last about 1 second and should result in visible chest rise. Avoid over-inflating the lungs.

6. Monitor and Adjust

- **Observe Chest Rise**: Ensure that each breath results in adequate chest rise. If not, adjust the mask position or head tilt.
- **Check for Airway Obstruction**: If there is no chest rise, recheck the airway for obstructions and adjust the mask or head position.

7. Perform CPR if Necessary

- **Combine with Chest Compressions**: If the patient is in cardiac arrest, continue chest compressions at a rate of 100-120 compressions per minute while using the BVM for ventilation.
- **Switch Roles**: If working with a team, switch roles with another responder to avoid fatigue and maintain effective CPR.

8. Prepare for Advanced Care

- **Prepare for Transfer**: Continue to provide BVM ventilation and support until advanced medical help arrives.
- **Communicate with Advanced Providers**: Provide a clear handoff to advanced care providers, detailing the patient's condition and the interventions performed.

Important Considerations

- **Proper Fit**: Ensure the mask fits well to avoid leaks. Adjust as needed to achieve a better seal.

- **Avoid Over-Ventilation:** Deliver breaths at a rate of about 10-12 breaths per minute for adults, and adjust based on patient needs and response.
- **Use of Supplemental Oxygen:** If using supplemental oxygen, adjust the flow rate according to protocols or guidelines.

Mastering the use of a BVM is essential for providing effective ventilation and improving the chances of survival in emergency situations.

Using oxygen equipment in Basic Life Support (BLS) involves several key steps to ensure proper administration and effective oxygen delivery. Here's a general overview:

Equipment

1. **Oxygen Cylinder:** Contains compressed oxygen.
2. **Regulator:** Controls the flow rate of oxygen.
3. **Oxygen Mask or Nasal Cannula:** Delivers oxygen to the patient.

Steps to Use Oxygen Equipment

1. **Check the Equipment:**
   - Ensure the oxygen cylinder is full and the regulator is properly attached.
   - Check for any visible damage to the equipment.
2. **Prepare the Regulator:**
   - Open the oxygen cylinder valve slowly to allow the regulator to adjust to the pressure.
   - Set the flow rate on the regulator as recommended (usually 2-6 liters per minute for nasal cannula or 10-15 liters per minute for a non-rebreather mask).
3. **Attach the Delivery Device:**
   - For a **Nasal Cannula:** Place the cannula prongs in the patient's nostrils and secure the tubing around the patient's ears.
   - For an **Oxygen Mask:** Position the mask over the patient's nose and mouth, ensuring a snug fit. Secure the straps around the patient's head.

4. **Adjust the Flow Rate:**
   - Ensure the flow rate is set according to the patient's needs and the type of delivery device used. For nasal cannulas, start with 2-4 liters per minute, and for masks, 10-15 liters per minute is common.
5. **Monitor the Patient:**
   - Continuously observe the patient for signs of improvement or distress.
   - Make sure the oxygen delivery device remains in place and is functioning correctly.
6. **Handle the Equipment Properly:**
   - Do not drop or shake the oxygen cylinder.
   - Keep the cylinder away from flammable materials.
7. **Document and Report:**
   - Record the oxygen therapy provided, including flow rates and duration, in the patient's documentation.
   - Report any changes in the patient's condition to the appropriate medical personnel.

Important Notes

- Always follow your local protocols and guidelines for oxygen administration.
- Ensure that you're trained and familiar with the specific oxygen equipment and procedures used in your setting.

Using a suction device on a patient is a critical skill for clearing the airway and ensuring proper breathing. Here's a step-by-step guide on how to use a suction device safely and effectively:

Equipment

1. **Suction Unit:** Portable or wall-mounted.
2. **Suction Catheter:** Appropriate size for the patient's airway (e.g., pediatric or adult).
3. **Collection Canister:** To collect the suctioned material.
4. **Suction Tubing:** Connects the catheter to the suction unit.
5. **Personal Protective Equipment (PPE):** Gloves, mask, and eye protection.

Steps for Using a Suction Device

1. **Preparation:**
   - **Assess the Situation:** Ensure suction is needed (e.g., visible secretions, noisy breathing).
   - **Prepare Equipment:** Check the suction device to ensure it is functioning correctly. Attach the suction catheter to the suction tubing and connect it to the suction unit.
   - **Wear PPE:** Put on gloves, a mask, and eye protection to prevent exposure to bodily fluids.
2. **Position the Patient:**
   - **For Conscious Patients:** Position them in a semi-sitting or upright position if possible. This helps prevent aspiration.
   - **For Unconscious or Semi-Conscious Patients:** Place them in the recovery position or lateral recumbent position to minimize the risk of aspiration.
3. **Suction Procedure:**
   - **Pre-oxygenate** (if applicable): Provide supplemental oxygen to the patient before suctioning if they are at high risk of hypoxia.
   - **Insert the Catheter:** Gently insert the suction catheter into the patient's airway. Avoid touching the back of the throat or the trachea to minimize gagging and irritation.
   - **Apply Suction:** Once the catheter is in the airway, apply suction by turning on the suction unit. Use intermittent suctioning (suction while withdrawing the catheter) to avoid damaging the airway and causing discomfort.
   - **Suction Time:** Limit suctioning to 10-15 seconds at a time to reduce the risk of hypoxia and trauma.
4. **Clear the Catheter:**
   - **Rinse the Catheter:** After suctioning, rinse the catheter with sterile water or saline to clear any debris. Dispose of or clean the catheter according to protocols.
   - **Recheck the Patient:** Assess the patient's airway and breathing. If needed, suction again or provide additional airway management.
5. **Document and Report:**

- **Record**: Document the amount and type of secretions, the duration of suctioning, and the patient's response.
- **Report**: Inform other healthcare providers of the patient's condition and any significant findings.

Important Considerations

- **Suction Pressure**: Adjust the suction pressure according to the patient's size and the type of suction device (typically between 80-120 mmHg for adults).
- **Frequency**: Avoid excessive suctioning to prevent irritation and damage to the airway.
- **Safety**: Always ensure proper hygiene and infection control practices to prevent cross-contamination.

Using a pulse oximeter in Basic Life Support (BLS) is a straightforward process. This device measures the oxygen saturation level in the blood and the pulse rate, providing valuable information about a patient's respiratory and circulatory status. Here's how to use it:

Equipment

1. **Pulse Oximeter**: Portable device with a probe.
2. **Sensor Probe**: Typically a clip-style probe for fingers, toes, or earlobes.

Steps for Using a Pulse Oximeter

1. **Prepare the Equipment:**
   - Ensure the pulse oximeter is in good working condition with fresh batteries if necessary.
2. **Position the Patient:**
   - **For Conscious Patients**: Position them comfortably. Make sure their hand or other site is still and relaxed.
   - **For Unconscious Patients**: Ensure that the probe can be attached securely, often on a finger, toe, or earlobe.
3. **Attach the Sensor Probe:**

- **Choose the Site**: Common sites include the fingertip, toe, or earlobe. For patients with poor peripheral circulation, use a site with better blood flow.
- **Place the Probe**: Attach the probe snugly to the chosen site. Ensure it is placed correctly for an accurate reading but avoid excessive tightness.

4. **Check the Reading**:
   - **Turn On the Device**: Power up the pulse oximeter. The display should show the oxygen saturation (SpO2) and pulse rate.
   - **Wait for Stable Readings**: Allow a few seconds for the device to stabilize and provide an accurate reading.

5. **Interpret the Results**:
   - **Oxygen Saturation (SpO2)**: Normal levels typically range from 95% to 100%. Values below 90% may indicate hypoxemia and warrant further intervention.
   - **Pulse Rate**: This should be consistent with the patient's normal range. Abnormal rates may indicate cardiovascular issues.

6. **Remove the Probe**:
   - Once you have obtained the readings, gently remove the probe from the patient's site.

7. **Document and Report**:
   - **Record**: Note the SpO2 and pulse rate readings in the patient's documentation.
   - **Report**: Inform other healthcare providers of the patient's oxygen saturation and pulse rate, especially if readings are abnormal.

Important Considerations

- **Accuracy**: Ensure the probe is well-positioned and that the patient is still. Movement, nail polish, or poor circulation can affect accuracy.
- **Calibration**: Regularly check the pulse oximeter for calibration and maintenance to ensure reliable readings.

- **Patient Factors:** Be aware of conditions that might affect readings, such as cold extremities, severe hypovolemia, or certain types of jaundice.

Using a pulse oximeter effectively helps you monitor the patient's respiratory and cardiovascular status, guiding further interventions in BLS.

Using a blood pressure cuff and stethoscope effectively is essential for accurate blood pressure measurement. Here's a step-by-step guide:

Equipment

1. **Blood Pressure Cuff:** Includes an inflatable bladder and a pressure gauge.
2. **Stethoscope:** For auscultation of the blood flow sounds.
3. **Sphygmomanometer:** The gauge that measures the pressure (often integrated with the cuff).

Steps for Measuring Blood Pressure

1. **Prepare the Patient:**
    - **Position:** Ensure the patient is seated comfortably with their back supported, feet flat on the floor, and arm at heart level.
    - **Rest:** Have the patient rest for at least 5 minutes before taking the measurement.
2. **Select the Cuff Size:**
    - **Size:** Use a cuff that fits the patient's arm appropriately. The bladder of the cuff should cover about 80% of the arm circumference.
3. **Position the Cuff:**
    - **Placement:** Place the cuff on the upper arm, about 1 inch above the elbow crease. Ensure it is snug but not too tight.
4. **Locate the Brachial Artery:**
    - **Palpate:** Feel for the brachial artery in the inner aspect of the arm, just above the elbow crease.
5. **Place the Stethoscope:**

- **Position:** Place the stethoscope's diaphragm over the brachial artery where you palpated it. Ensure a good seal to hear the sounds clearly.

6. **Inflate the Cuff:**
   - **Pump Up:** Inflate the cuff by squeezing the bulb. Continue inflating until the gauge reads about 20-30 mmHg above the expected systolic pressure (usually around 180 mmHg for most adults).

7. **Deflate the Cuff Slowly:**
   - **Open the Valve:** Slowly release the pressure by turning the valve on the bulb. Deflate at a rate of about 2-3 mmHg per second.

8. **Listen and Record:**
   - **Systolic Pressure:** Note the reading on the gauge when you first hear the rhythmic tapping sounds (Korotkoff sounds). This is the systolic pressure.
   - **Diastolic Pressure:** Continue to listen as the tapping sounds become muffled and eventually disappear. The point where the sound disappears is the diastolic pressure.

9. **Complete the Measurement:**
   - **Remove the Cuff:** Once the measurement is complete, fully deflate and remove the cuff.
   - **Record the Results:** Document the systolic and diastolic pressures. The reading is recorded as "systolic/diastolic" (e.g., 120/80 mmHg).

Tips for Accurate Measurement

- **Arm Position:** The arm should be relaxed and supported at heart level.
- **Cuff Fit:** Ensure the cuff is properly fitted. A cuff that is too small or too large can result in inaccurate readings.
- **Patient Movement:** The patient should remain still and quiet during the measurement.
- **Repeat Measurements:** If necessary, take multiple readings and average them for a more accurate result.

By following these steps, you can ensure accurate and reliable blood pressure measurements. If you have any more questions or specific scenarios, let me know!

Applying trauma dressing and bandages is crucial for managing bleeding and protecting wounds. Here's a step-by-step guide on how to do it effectively:

1. Assess the Situation

- **Evaluate the Wound**: Determine the severity of the wound and the extent of bleeding.
- **Ensure Safety**: Make sure the environment is safe for you and the patient.

2. Gather Supplies

- **Sterile Dressings**: Gauze pads, trauma dressings, or sterile bandages.
- **Adhesive Tape or Bandages**: To secure the dressing.
- **Antiseptic** (if applicable): For cleaning the wound.
- **Gloves**: To protect yourself and the patient.

3. Prepare the Wound

- **Wear Gloves**: Protect yourself from potential infection.
- **Clean the Wound**: If possible, gently clean the wound with sterile water or saline. Avoid using antiseptic solutions directly in deep wounds.
- **Control Bleeding**: Apply gentle pressure directly on the wound to control bleeding before applying the dressing.

4. Apply the Dressing

- **Choose the Dressing**: Select an appropriate size and type of dressing based on the wound.
- **Place the Dressing**: Lay the sterile dressing over the wound, ensuring it covers the entire area.

- **Apply Pressure**: If the wound is bleeding heavily, apply additional pressure with a gauze pad or trauma dressing.

5. Secure the Dressing

- **Use Adhesive Tape or Bandage**: Secure the dressing in place with adhesive tape or a bandage. Ensure it is snug but not too tight to avoid cutting off circulation.
- **Wrap the Bandage**: If using a bandage, start wrapping from the distal end of the limb (farther from the body) and move towards the proximal end (closer to the body). Ensure that the bandage is evenly applied without gaps.

6. Check for Circulation

- **Assess Circulation**: After securing the dressing, check the extremity for signs of good circulation, such as warmth, color, and pulse. Ensure that the bandage is not too tight and does not impair circulation.

7. Monitor and Reassess

- **Monitor the Wound**: Continuously check the wound and dressing for signs of worsening or additional bleeding.
- **Reapply if Necessary**: If the dressing becomes saturated or the bleeding continues, replace the dressing with a new one. Apply additional dressings as needed, always maintaining pressure.

8. Document and Seek Further Care

- **Record Details**: Document the type of dressing used, the condition of the wound, and any other relevant information.
- **Seek Professional Help**: Arrange for the patient to receive further medical evaluation and treatment as needed.

Additional Tips

- **For Large Wounds**: Use a larger dressing or multiple dressings to cover the wound completely.

- **For Embedded Objects**: Do not remove objects that are embedded in the wound. Stabilize the object with dressings and seek professional medical help.
- **For Burns**: Cover burns with a sterile non-stick dressing and avoid using adhesive tape directly on the burn.

Effective trauma dressing and bandaging can help control bleeding, reduce the risk of infection, and protect the wound until professional medical treatment is available.

Using splints in Basic Life Support (BLS) is essential for immobilizing and stabilizing injured limbs to prevent further injury and reduce pain. Here's a step-by-step guide on how to use splints effectively:

Equipment

1. **Splints**: Rigid or semi-rigid materials, such as commercial splints, padded boards, or improvised splints (e.g., rolled-up newspapers).
2. **Padding**: Soft material like gauze or cloth to cushion the splint.
3. **Bandages or Straps**: To secure the splint in place.

Steps for Applying a Splint

1. **Assess the Situation**
   - **Check the Injury**: Determine the location and severity of the injury. Look for signs of fractures, dislocations, or severe sprains.
   - **Ensure Safety**: Make sure the scene is safe and that you and the patient are not in immediate danger.
2. **Prepare the Patient**
   - **Comfort**: Position the patient comfortably. Avoid moving the injured area unnecessarily.
   - **Assess Circulation**: Check for pulses, color, and temperature of the injured limb before applying the splint. This helps identify any pre-existing circulation issues.
3. **Apply Padding**

- **Protect the Skin**: Place padding around the injured area to prevent pressure sores and reduce discomfort. Ensure the padding covers any bony areas or open wounds.

4. **Select and Position the Splint**
   - **Choose a Splint**: Use an appropriate-sized splint for the injury. If a commercial splint is unavailable, use an improvised splint that is rigid and stable.
   - **Align the Injury**: Gently align the injured limb to its normal position. Avoid realigning the bones if they are displaced or protruding.
5. **Apply the Splint**
   - **Place the Splint**: Position the splint on either side of the injured limb. Ensure it extends beyond the joints above and below the injury to immobilize the entire limb.
   - **Secure the Splint**: Use bandages, straps, or cloth to secure the splint in place. Wrap the bandages or straps snugly but not too tight. Avoid cutting off circulation.
6. **Recheck Circulation**
   - **Assess**: After securing the splint, check the limb for circulation. Ensure that the fingers or toes remain warm, pink, and that pulses are present.
   - **Adjust if Necessary**: If circulation is impaired, loosen the bandages or straps slightly to restore blood flow.
7. **Monitor and Comfort**
   - **Reassess**: Continuously monitor the patient for any changes in their condition. Provide comfort and reassurance.
   - **Documentation**: Record details about the injury, the type of splint used, and the patient's response to the splinting.
8. **Seek Medical Attention**
   - **Arrange for Transport**: Ensure the patient receives appropriate medical evaluation and treatment as soon as possible. Call for emergency medical services if necessary.

Additional Tips

- **Avoid Movement**: Minimize movement of the injured limb during splinting to prevent further injury.

- **Improvised Splints**: In emergencies, you can use rigid objects like boards, rolled-up newspapers, or magazines as makeshift splints.
- **Splinting Fractures**: For suspected fractures, apply the splint above and below the fracture site. Do not attempt to realign bone fragments.

Proper splinting helps stabilize the injury, reduce pain, and prevent further complications. If you have specific questions or scenarios, feel free to ask!

Applying airway management tools in Basic Life Support (BLS) involves using devices and techniques to ensure that a patient's airway is clear and unobstructed, allowing for adequate breathing. Here's how to use common airway management tools effectively:

1. Basic Airway Management

Head-Tilt, Chin-Lift Maneuver

- **Purpose**: To open the airway in an unconscious patient by lifting the tongue away from the back of the throat.
- **Steps**:
    1. **Position the Patient**: Place the patient on their back.
    2. **Perform the Maneuver**: Place one hand on the patient's forehead and apply gentle pressure to tilt the head back. With your other hand, lift the chin forward. Ensure the airway is open.

Jaw-Thrust Maneuver

- **Purpose**: To open the airway without extending the neck, useful for patients with suspected spinal injuries.
- **Steps**:
    1. **Position the Patient**: Place the patient on their back.
    2. **Perform the Maneuver**: Place your fingers behind the angles of the jaw and lift the jaw upward, while using your thumbs to push down on the patient's lower lip. Ensure the airway is open.

2. Oropharyngeal Airway (OPA)

Purpose: To keep the airway open by preventing the tongue from obstructing it in unconscious patients.

Steps:

1. **Measure the OPA**: Choose the correct size by measuring from the patient's earlobe to the corner of the mouth.
2. **Position the Patient**: Place the patient on their back.
3. **Insert the OPA**:
    - **Align**: Hold the OPA with the curved side facing up and insert it into the mouth.
    - **Rotate**: Gently rotate the OPA 180 degrees as you advance it into the airway. This helps the tip to avoid the soft palate and tongue.
    - **Secure**: Ensure the OPA is positioned properly and does not obstruct the airway or cause discomfort.

3. Nasopharyngeal Airway (NPA)

Purpose: To provide an airway in patients who are conscious or semi-conscious and where an OPA might be inappropriate.

Steps:

1. **Measure the NPA**: Choose the correct size by measuring from the patient's nostril to the earlobe.
2. **Position the Patient**: Place the patient on their back.
3. **Insert the NPA**:
    - **Lubricate**: Apply a water-based lubricant to the NPA.
    - **Insert**: Gently insert the NPA into the patient's nostril, aiming towards the ear.
    - **Advance**: Continue advancing the NPA until the flange rests against the nostril. Do not force it.

4. Bag-Valve-Mask (BVM) Ventilation

Purpose: To provide positive pressure ventilation for patients who are not breathing or have inadequate breathing.

Steps:

1. **Position the Patient**: Place the patient on their back.
2. **Seal the Mask**: Place the mask over the patient's nose and mouth. Use the E-C clamp technique: place the heel of one hand on the mask to create a seal, and use your fingers to hold the mandible (lower jaw) up.
3. **Attach the Bag**: Connect the BVM to the oxygen source if available.
4. **Ventilate**: Squeeze the bag gently to deliver air into the patient's lungs. Watch for chest rise and listen for breath sounds. Ensure the mask is properly sealed and the airway is clear.

5. Endotracheal Intubation (Advanced Skill, typically beyond basic BLS scope)

Purpose: To secure the airway in patients who cannot be managed with basic techniques. This involves placing an endotracheal tube into the trachea.

Steps:

1. **Prepare the Equipment**: Assemble the intubation kit, including the endotracheal tube and laryngoscope.
2. **Position the Patient**: Place the patient in the "sniffing" position (head tilted slightly back).
3. **Insert the Laryngoscope**: Use the laryngoscope to visualize the vocal cords.
4. **Insert the Endotracheal Tube**: Advance the tube through the vocal cords into the trachea.
5. **Verify Placement**: Confirm tube placement by auscultating the lungs and checking for chest rise.

General Tips

- **Monitor the Patient:** Continuously check the patient's breathing and oxygenation status.
- **Proper Technique:** Ensure that all airway devices are used according to protocol to avoid complications.
- **Seek Help:** If you are unsure or the patient's condition deteriorates, seek advanced medical assistance.

Using these airway management tools effectively helps to maintain a clear airway and ensure adequate breathing, which is crucial in emergency situations.

The "enroute to hospital" process in Basic Life Support (BLS) involves managing and monitoring the patient while they are being transported to a medical facility. Here's a step-by-step guide on how to handle this crucial phase:

1. Initial Assessment and Stabilization

- **Primary Survey:** Quickly assess the patient's airway, breathing, circulation, and level of consciousness. Address any immediate life threats.
- **Stabilize:** Implement appropriate interventions, such as CPR, airway management, or bleeding control, based on the patient's condition.

2. Prepare for Transport

- **Hand Over to EMS:** If emergency medical services (EMS) are arriving, provide a concise and accurate handover, including the patient's condition, interventions performed, and any changes in their status.
- **Documentation:** Record all relevant information, including vital signs, treatments administered, and any observations.

3. Monitor the Patient

- **Vital Signs:** Continuously monitor and record vital signs, such as heart rate, blood pressure, respiratory rate, and oxygen saturation.

- **Comfort and Reassurance**: Keep the patient comfortable and provide reassurance if they are conscious. Address any concerns or discomfort they might have.

4. Provide Ongoing Care

- **Airway Management**: Ensure that the airway remains open and clear. Continue to use airway management tools as necessary.
- **CPR**: If performing CPR, ensure compressions and ventilations are effective and adjust as needed based on the patient's response.
- **Fluid and Medication**: If applicable, manage intravenous fluids or medications according to protocols.

5. Communicate with the Receiving Facility

- **Alert the Hospital**: If possible, communicate with the receiving hospital to provide a report on the patient's condition and estimated time of arrival. This allows the hospital to prepare for the patient's arrival.
- **Provide Information**: Give a detailed handover to hospital staff upon arrival, including patient history, treatments provided, and current status.

6. Ensure Safe Transport

- **Secure the Patient**: Ensure the patient is safely secured on the stretcher or transport vehicle. Avoid unnecessary movement that could worsen their condition.
- **Monitor Environment**: Be aware of the transport environment, including any potential hazards or changes that could affect the patient's condition.

7. Handle Complications

- **Respond to Changes**: Be prepared to handle any changes or complications that arise during transport, such as deterioration in the patient's condition or new symptoms.

- **Adjust Care**: Modify your interventions as needed based on the patient's evolving condition and the guidance of medical protocols.

8. Post-Arrival

- **Assist with Transfer**: Help with transferring the patient to the hospital's care, ensuring a smooth handover to the hospital staff.
- **Complete Documentation**: Ensure all relevant documentation is completed, including patient care records and any incident reports.

Key Considerations

- **Stay Calm**: Maintaining a calm demeanor helps in managing both the patient and any accompanying family members or bystanders.
- **Follow Protocols**: Adhere to established protocols and guidelines for patient care and transport.
- **Safety**: Prioritize patient safety throughout the transport process, including monitoring for signs of complications and addressing them promptly.

Effective management during the enroute phase is critical to ensuring that the patient arrives at the hospital in the best possible condition for further treatment.

The handover process in Basic Life Support (BLS) is crucial for ensuring continuity of care when transferring a patient to another healthcare provider, such as emergency medical services (EMS) or hospital staff. A clear and comprehensive handover helps ensure that all necessary information is communicated effectively. Here's a detailed guide on how to perform a handover in BLS:

1. Prepare for Handover

- **Gather Information**: Collect all relevant patient information, including vital signs, treatments administered, and the patient's response to interventions.

- **Organize Documentation**: Ensure that all documentation is complete and accurate, including patient records, treatment logs, and any incident reports.

2. Provide a Clear and Concise Report

When handing over to EMS or hospital staff, follow a structured approach to ensure all critical information is communicated:

Patient Identification

- **Name and Age**: Provide the patient's full name and age.
- **Identification Details**: Include any identification numbers or relevant personal details.

Chief Complaint and History

- **Reason for Call**: Summarize the primary reason for the emergency or the patient's chief complaint.
- **Medical History**: Briefly describe relevant medical history, including chronic conditions, allergies, and medications.

Current Condition

- **Vital Signs**: Report the most recent vital signs, such as heart rate, blood pressure, respiratory rate, and oxygen saturation.
- **Level of Consciousness**: Describe the patient's level of consciousness (e.g., alert, drowsy, unresponsive).

Interventions and Treatments

- **Actions Taken**: Detail any interventions performed, such as CPR, airway management, or bleeding control.
- **Medications and Fluids**: Provide information on any medications administered or intravenous fluids given.
- **Response to Treatment**: Explain how the patient has responded to the interventions.

Physical Exam Findings

- **Injuries and Symptoms**: Describe any visible injuries, symptoms, or abnormalities found during the assessment.
- **Additional Observations**: Note any changes in the patient's condition, such as worsening symptoms or improvement.

Special Considerations

- **Allergies and Reactions**: Mention any known allergies or adverse reactions observed.
- **Family Concerns**: If applicable, include any concerns or requests from family members.

3. Communicate Effectively

- **Use Clear Language**: Avoid medical jargon and use plain language to ensure that all information is easily understood.
- **Be Concise**: Provide essential information without unnecessary detail, focusing on what is most relevant to the patient's care.
- **Encourage Questions**: Allow the receiving provider to ask questions and clarify any uncertainties.

4. Assist with Transfer

- **Patient Transfer**: Ensure that the patient is safely and comfortably transferred to the care of EMS or hospital staff.
- **Confirm Receipt**: Verify that the receiving team has received and understood the handover information.
- **Provide Documentation**: Share any written documentation or records with the receiving provider as needed.

5. Document the Handover

- **Record Details**: Document the details of the handover, including the time, names of the receiving personnel, and any specific instructions or concerns communicated.
- **Review Documentation**: Ensure all patient records and handover notes are complete and accurate.

Key Considerations

- **Confidentiality:** Maintain patient confidentiality throughout the handover process.
- **Timeliness:** Conduct the handover in a timely manner to minimize delays in patient care.
- **Continuity of Care:** Ensure that the information provided supports a seamless transition and ongoing patient management.

Effective handover is vital for ensuring that the patient receives appropriate care throughout their treatment journey.

A Basic Life Support (BLS) course for paramedics is essential for ensuring that healthcare providers have the skills and knowledge required to manage life-threatening emergencies effectively. Here's a conclusion summarizing the key aspects of such a course:

Conclusion on Paramedic Basic Life Support Course

1. **Core Competencies:**
   - **Assessment Skills:** Paramedics learn to rapidly assess and prioritize life-threatening conditions, including airway obstruction, cardiac arrest, and severe bleeding.
   - **Intervention Techniques:** The course covers critical BLS techniques, including CPR, airway management, and the use of automated external defibrillators (AEDs).
   - **Patient Management:** Emphasis is placed on effective patient management during emergencies, including the use of splints, bandages, and other first aid measures.
2. **Practical Application:**
   - **Hands-On Training:** Practical exercises and simulations help paramedics develop and refine their skills in a controlled environment, enhancing their ability to perform under real-life conditions.
   - **Scenario-Based Learning:** Participants engage in scenario-based training to apply theoretical knowledge to practical situations, improving their decision-making and problem-solving abilities.
3. **Standards and Protocols:**
   - **Adherence to Guidelines:** The course ensures that paramedics are familiar with and adhere to current

guidelines and protocols for BLS, including those from organizations such as the American Heart Association (AHA) or equivalent bodies.
- **Consistency in Care**: Training fosters consistency in delivering high-quality care, reducing variability and improving patient outcomes in emergency situations.

4. **Communication and Teamwork**:
   - **Effective Handover**: Emphasis is placed on the importance of clear and concise communication during patient handovers to ensure continuity of care.
   - **Collaborative Skills**: Paramedics learn to work effectively as part of a team, coordinating with other healthcare providers to deliver comprehensive care.

5. **Ongoing Education and Improvement**:
   - **Continual Learning**: The course highlights the need for ongoing education and skill maintenance to keep up with advances in emergency care and best practices.
   - **Self-Assessment**: Paramedics are encouraged to continuously assess and improve their skills through regular training and review.

6. **Patient-Centered Approach**:
   - **Safety and Comfort**: Paramedics are trained to prioritize patient safety and comfort while performing life-saving interventions.
   - **Compassionate Care**: The course emphasizes the importance of providing compassionate care to patients and their families during high-stress situations.

Summary

A Basic Life Support course for paramedics is crucial for equipping healthcare providers with the essential skills to manage emergencies effectively. Through a combination of theoretical knowledge, practical training, and adherence to established protocols, paramedics are prepared to provide high-quality care, improve patient outcomes, and work collaboratively in emergency situations. Ongoing education and a patient-centered approach further enhance their ability to deliver effective and compassionate care.